AI for Nurses

The Practical Guide to HIPAA Compliant AI Tools, Documentation Workflows, and Ethical Integration for Registered Nurses and Nurse Practitioners

Arrow Jay Publishing

This book is intended for educational purposes only. The information contained herein does not constitute medical, legal, or compliance advice. Nurses should follow their facility's policies, their state's nursing practice act, and all applicable regulatory requirements when integrating AI tools into their practice. The authors and publisher disclaim any liability arising from the use or misuse of the information in this book.

AI for Nurses is part of the AI for Professionals Series.

ISBN (Paperback): 978-1-964326-07-8

ISBN (eBook): 978-1-964326-10-8

First Edition, 2026

Important Notice

This book is designed to provide practical guidance for registered nurses and nurse practitioners considering the integration of artificial intelligence tools into their clinical documentation workflows. It is intended for educational purposes only.

Nothing in this book constitutes medical, legal, or compliance advice. The authors and publisher strongly recommend that nurses:

- Consult their facility's compliance and informatics teams before adopting any AI tool for clinical use
- Review their state's nursing practice act and any applicable licensure regulations
- Obtain guidance from their professional organization regarding AI integration in their specialty
- Verify HIPAA compliance of any tool before using it with patient-adjacent information

The AI landscape evolves rapidly. Specific tools, policies, and regulations referenced in this book reflect information available as of the publication date and may have changed. Always verify current information from authoritative sources.

The nurse retains full professional and legal accountability for all clinical documentation, regardless of the tools used in its preparation.

A Note on AI-Assisted Writing: This book was researched, structured, and written with the assistance of AI tools. All content has been reviewed, edited, and approved by the publisher. The use of AI in the preparation of this manuscript is consistent with the principles described throughout this book, that AI is a productivity tool that amplifies human judgment, not a replacement for it.

Introduction

There is a moment most nurses know.

The shift has ended. The night team is at the station. Your patients are covered. And you are still there, in front of a screen, documenting everything that happened in the past twelve hours. The hallway is quiet. The parking lot is dark. Somewhere between the assessment findings and the care plan updates, you wonder how this became the job.

It was not supposed to be like this. You went to nursing school to be with patients, to be the person in the room when something matters, to do the clinical work that keeps people safe and helps them heal. The documentation was always part of it, but it was supposed to be the record of care, not the destination of care.

For many nurses in 2026, documentation has become the destination. Hours at a keyboard for every hour at the bedside. Notes written after the shift, in the car, at midnight, from memory. Documentation has become a burden. It reduces the time nurses have to spend with patients, and it is one of the most significant drivers of the burnout crisis. This burden is taking nurses out of the workforce faster than the system can replace them.

This book exists because something changed. Not the documentation requirements. Not the staffing ratios. Not the healthcare system. What changed is that there is now a practical, accessible tool that can take the structural work of documentation off your hands and give you something back.

AI for Nurses is the practical guide to using that tool safely, ethically, and effectively. It covers every step from understanding the legal and ethical framework to writing your first prompt to building documentation habits that will carry you through your career. It was written for registered nurses and nurse practitioners in every setting, from the ICU to home health, from new graduates to experienced nurses who have been doing this for decades.

This is not a book about technology. It is a book about using technology to reclaim the time and energy that administrative work has been taking from you.

How to Use This Book

If you are new to AI and want to understand the landscape before doing anything, read Chapters 1 through 3 first. If you are ready to start writing prompts, go to Chapters 4 and 5, then Chapter 6 for the workflow guide. If you want to get started immediately, go to the Quick Start section, then return to the foundational chapters when you have time.

If you are a nurse leader or educator using this book to support your team, Chapter 12 on implementation and Chapter 13 on case studies will be the most directly applicable starting points. The prompt library in Appendix A is designed to be used from day one.

Contents

Quick Start: Your First 30 Minutes with AI

This section is for the nurse who wants to get started today. Come back and read the full book when you have time. For the next thirty minutes, here is exactly what to do.

Step 1: Choose Your Tool (5 Minutes)

If your facility has an approved clinical AI tool, use that. If not, you can use a general AI tool for the non-patient-specific tasks in this Quick Start. No patient information will be involved in the next thirty minutes.

Step 2: Write Your First Prompt (10 Minutes)

Open your AI tool. Type or paste this prompt:

PROMPT: You are a registered nurse preparing a patient education handout. Write a simple one-page guide for a patient going home after being diagnosed with high blood pressure for the first time. Use a 6th grade reading level. Include: what high blood pressure is in plain language, three lifestyle changes the patient can make, information about taking medication as prescribed, and when to call the doctor. Use short paragraphs. End with a brief checklist the patient can use at home.

Read what comes back. Notice how specific the prompt is and how specific the output is. Now modify it slightly. Change the condition to something common in your practice area. Submit again and compare the two outputs.

Step 3: Try a Handoff Summary (10 Minutes)

Using a fictional patient with no real information, try this prompt:

PROMPT: You are a registered nurse preparing an end-of-shift SBAR handoff summary. Write an SBAR for a fictional 65-year-old male patient admitted with pneumonia. He is on day 2 of antibiotics, vital signs are stable, oxygen requirement has decreased from 4L nasal cannula to 2L over the past 24 hours, he ambulated in the hallway this morning, he has a productive cough and is on scheduled cough medication. Use standard SBAR format.

Read the output. Is it structured? Is it complete? What would you add if this were a real patient?

Step 4: Save Your First Prompts (5 Minutes)

Copy both prompts into a document, a note on your phone, or wherever you keep working notes. Label them clearly. You just started your .personal prompt library.

Chapter 1
Introduction to AI in Nursing Practice

Maria Santos finished charting at 11:47 PM.

Her shift had ended at 7. She had spent the first forty minutes giving a report to the night nurse, answered two call lights that could not wait, and then sat down at the nursing station to do what she always did after a twelve-hour shift: document everything she had done for the past twelve hours.

Four patients. One admitted mid-shift with chest pain who required continuous monitoring, frequent reassessment, and a cascade of orders she had to track and execute. One preparing for discharge who needed teaching on her new blood thinner, her fall risk precautions, and when to call her cardiologist. One who had been stable all day until 4 PM, when his oxygen saturation started trending in the wrong direction and Maria spent ninety minutes managing the response. One straightforward post-op recovery who still required hourly assessments and pain documentation.

Four patients. Nearly five hours of charting.

She drove home in the dark, too tired to be hungry, too wired to sleep. She sat in her car in the driveway for a few minutes before going inside, running back through the shift. She wondered, did she document everything correctly? Had she missed anything in the new admission's assessment? Had she been clear enough in her handoff about the oxygen situation?

This is nursing in 2026. And this is why this book exists.

The Documentation Burden in Real Numbers

The nursing profession has a burnout problem that everyone recognizes. According to the National Council of State Boards of Nursing 2024 Workforce Study, more than 138,000 nurses left the workforce between 2022 and 2024. Almost 40 percent of currently practicing nurses report intent to leave the profession by 2029.

When nurses are asked directly why they are burned out, staffing ratios come up first. Then comes something that does not always make headlines: the paperwork. The charting. The documentation burden has grown steadily for two decades as electronic health records added fields, compliance requirements added layers, and reimbursement structures turned clinical encounters into coding exercises.

Research published in the American Nurse Journal places nursing documentation time at 25 to 40 percent of a full shift. Clinical workflow studies show an average of 2.5 hours per shift spent on documentation alone. If you are a nurse reading those numbers and thinking they feel conservative, you are probably right.

Documentation matters. Accurate, timely, complete charting protects patients, supports care coordination, enables billing, and documents the nursing process that keeps people alive. The argument is simpler than that: nurses should not be spending nearly half their professional time writing about care at the expense of actually providing it.

The 2026 Landscape: Where AI and Nursing Meet

Artificial intelligence has been present in healthcare for years. The sepsis alert that fires in your EHR when a patient's vitals trend in a dangerous direction. The early warning score that flags deterioration risk. The medication interaction check that happens automatically when a provider enters an order. These are AI systems, and they have been saving lives quietly for more than a decade.

What changed in the last two to three years is different. The emergence of large language models, the type of AI behind tools like ChatGPT, Claude, and Gemini, created something new: AI that can read text, understand context, and write clinically appropriate language. Suddenly the thing that consumed most of a nurse's non-bedside time became something AI could help with.

A 2025 peer-reviewed study published in Nursing Open found that AI integration in clinical settings reduced nursing documentation time from approximately 15 minutes to 5 minutes per entry. Hospitals piloting AI-powered documentation tools report significant reductions in charting time alongside improved nurse satisfaction. The American Hospital Association noted in 2025 that AI advances in nursing documentation are receiving serious institutional attention for the first time.

The AI for Professionals Series exists to close the gap between what is possible and what is actually happening at the bedside. This book is the nursing edition. It was written for the nurse who has heard that AI can help with documentation but does not know how to start, what tools are safe, what the legal and ethical issues are, or whether the promise is real. It was written for the nurse practitioner who spends evenings catching up on notes when she could be sleeping. It was written for the floor nurse who gives a silent sigh every time she opens the charting screen after a twelve-hour shift.

What AI Can and Cannot Do in Nursing Practice

Before going further, it is worth being precise about what AI can and cannot do. This matters not just for practical reasons, but because the misuse of AI in clinical settings has real consequences for patients and for nursing licenses.

Where AI Genuinely Helps

- Converting anonymized clinical bullet points into structured note formats such as SOAP, DAR, PIE, and Focus Charting
- Drafting patient education materials, handouts, medication teaching, and discharge instructions
- Preparing structured shift handoffs in SBAR format
- Supporting care planning by generating goal and intervention options for nurse review
- Assisting with nurse self-reflection and professional development documentation

What AI Cannot Do

- Assess your patient - it has no access to the room, no sensory input, no bedside intuition
- Replace clinical judgment - it cannot catch the subtle signs that tell you something is wrong
- Guarantee accuracy - language models produce plausible-sounding content that can be factually incorrect
- Accept responsibility - the license is yours, and accountability does not transfer to any tool

Addressing Common Concerns

The conversation about AI in nursing generates strong reactions in both directions, and most of them are based on incomplete information.

Will AI replace nurses? No. A language model cannot take a blood pressure, insert an IV, recognize the sound of labored breathing, hold a patient's hand, or make a judgment call in a deteriorating situation. What AI is replacing is the administrative burden that surrounds that work. If AI eliminates two hours of nightly charting, nursing becomes more nursing, not less.

Is using AI for documentation unethical? No. Using AI to help structure and draft clinical documentation is no different in principle from using a template, a macro, or a documentation assistant. The ethical question is whether the documentation accurately reflects your clinical assessment and whether you reviewed and approved it.

Is AI too complicated for clinical nurses? No. The basic workflow requires no technical background. You describe what happened, paste it into a compliant tool with a prompt, read what comes back, edit and approve. The prompt engineering skills in Chapters 4 and 5 deepen your capability over time, but the entry point is genuinely accessible.

Your Path Forward

Maria Santos would not hear about AI documentation tools for another four months after that night in her car. A colleague mentioned it during a break. She was skeptical, then curious, then methodical: she read about HIPAA compliance, found a tool with a signed Business Associate Agreement, practiced on a few notes, and started slowly.

Six months later she was charting on most nights before she left the unit. She still reviews every note. She still signs her name to every entry. She still catches things the AI missed or got wrong, and she corrects them. But she gets home before midnight now. She is less tired.

This book is the guide she would have wanted when she started.

End-of-Shift Handoff Pitfalls and How to Avoid Them

The most common failure in AI-assisted handoffs is not that the AI gets something wrong. It is that the nurse does not read the output carefully before using it. A handoff that sounds complete and professional is not the same as a handoff that is clinically accurate and complete. Speed is the enemy of review, and the end of a shift is exactly when speed is most tempting.

Three specific pitfalls appear consistently across nurses who have been using AI handoff tools for more than a few weeks. The first is accepting output that is structurally correct but missing qualitative observations. AI will organize what you give it, but it cannot add what you did not include. The nurse who noticed that a patient seemed more anxious than usual, that a family member was asking pointed questions about the plan of care, or that a wound looked slightly different than yesterday needs to add those observations manually. They will not appear in the AI output unless you put them in the prompt.

The second pitfall is using outdated notes as input. If you collect your shift notes at 2 PM for a 7 PM handoff, anything that changed in those five hours is missing from your prompt. Build the habit of adding a final note capture in the last thirty minutes of the shift, specifically to catch the changes that happened late.

The third pitfall is handing off the AI output verbally without reviewing it first. Some nurses generate the SBAR, give reports verbally while the output is on screen, and assume the two match. Read the output before you speak. Correct it before you hand it off. The incoming nurse is depending on that information to keep your patients safe.

Transfer Handoffs and Escalation Situations

Transfer handoffs, (moving a patient from one unit to another, from the ED to the floor, from the floor to the ICU) are among the highest-risk communication events in healthcare. Research consistently identifies transfer handoffs as a significant source of adverse events, near-misses, and information loss. The structured SBAR format is even more important in these situations than in routine end-of-shift handoffs, because the receiving nurse has no prior relationship with the patient and no context beyond what you provide.

AI-assisted transfer handoffs work best when the prompt explicitly calls out the transfer context. Include the reason for transfer, the clinical trajectory that led to the decision, any pending orders or results that the receiving unit will need to act on, family communication that has occurred and any outstanding family concerns, and specific information about the patient's baseline that would not be obvious from the chart alone.

For rapid response and escalation situations, the handoff requirements are different. Speed matters more than completeness, and the SBAR needs to convey the essential clinical picture in under two minutes. Keep a short rapid-response SBAR prompt saved on your phone, one that asks for situation and immediate clinical concern first, then fills in background and recommendations. The goal is not a comprehensive summary. It is getting the right person the right information fast enough to matter.

Prompt 9 in Appendix A is specifically designed for rapid response situations. Review it before you need it, not while you are in the middle of an emergency.

A Practical Workflow for High-Frequency Education Topics

Most nursing units have five to ten patient education topics that come up repeatedly. Post-operative care for the most common procedures in your unit. Medication teaching for the drugs most frequently prescribed at discharge. Management instructions for the chronic conditions most commonly seen in your patient population. These are the topics where building a prompt library pays off most quickly.

The workflow is straightforward. Identify your top five recurring education topics. For each one, draft a prompt that produces a solid first-draft handout. Refine the prompt over two or three uses until the output consistently requires minimal editing. Save that prompt. Now you have a library of five prompts that will save you meaningful time every shift.

Over time, this library grows. A nurse who has been using AI for patient education for six months typically has fifteen to twenty reliable prompts covering the most common situations in her practice. Each one represents a task that used to take fifteen to thirty minutes and now takes two to five minutes. The cumulative time savings across a career are significant.

The important discipline is not letting the library become a substitute for thinking. A prompt that reliably produces good output for a stable, literate adult patient may produce output that is entirely wrong for a patient with cognitive impairment, low health literacy, or a complex comorbidity profile. Always review output with the specific patient in mind, not the generic patient the prompt was written for.

Language Access and Working With Interpreters

Language access in patient education is a patient rights issue, not a courtesy. Patients with limited English proficiency have a federal right to receive health information in a language they can understand. In practice, nursing units rarely have adequate interpreted education materials for every patient who needs them, and nurses routinely improvise under time pressure with inadequate materials.

AI can meaningfully improve this situation with an important caveat. General AI tools can produce reasonable first-draft translations of patient education materials in many common languages. The quality varies significantly by language, and it is never sufficient to give a patient an AI-translated document without having it reviewed by a qualified interpreter or a bilingual clinical staff member who can verify accuracy.

The appropriate use is this: use AI to produce a draft translation that gives the interpreter a starting point to review and correct, rather than starting from scratch. This reduces the interpreter's time investment and makes it more likely that materials will actually be prepared and used. A qualified review step is not optional, it is a patient safety requirement.

For facilities with regular interpreter services, the workflow is: generate the AI draft, send it to the interpreter for review and correction before patient use, and document that reviewed materials were provided. For facilities where interpreter access is limited, work with your compliance or quality team to establish a review process before using AI-generated translated materials with patients.

Questions to Ask Before You Commit to Any Tool

Evaluating an AI tool for clinical use is different from evaluating a consumer app. The stakes are higher, the compliance requirements are specific, and the consequences of choosing wrong are not just inconvenience, they are potential HIPAA violations and patient safety risks. Before committing to any tool for clinical use, work through these questions.

On compliance: Does the vendor offer a Business Associate Agreement, and will they sign one with your organization? Where is patient data stored and in what jurisdiction? What is the vendor's breach notification policy and history? Has the tool been reviewed by your facility's security and compliance teams?

On data use: Does the vendor use your inputs to train their AI models? If so, can you opt out? What is the data retention policy? How long does the vendor store your inputs and outputs? Can you request deletion? These questions matter particularly for nurses in private practice or small clinic settings who may not have an institutional compliance team to consult.

On clinical fit: Was the tool designed for healthcare use or adapted from a general-purpose AI? Does it produce output in standard nursing documentation formats, (SOAP, DAR, SBAR) or does it require significant reformatting? Has it been validated in settings similar to yours? What do nurses in your specialty say about it?

On sustainability: What is the pricing model and how has it changed over the past year? Is the company financially stable? What happens to your data if the company is acquired or shuts down? These are not hypothetical concerns; the AI tool market is consolidating rapidly and tools that exist today may look very different in eighteen months.

Building the Case for Institutional Adoption

Many nurses reading this book are working in facilities that have not yet approved any AI documentation tools. If you are in that situation, you are not stuck, you can use the anonymization approach for non-PHI tasks while building the case for institutional adoption. Here is how to approach that conversation.

Lead with data, not enthusiasm. Estimate the documentation hours your unit spends per week and calculate what a 30 percent reduction would mean in nursing hours recovered. Frame this as a staffing and retention issue, because that is what it is. Nursing leadership and hospital administration respond to arguments about staffing capacity and retention far more readily than to arguments about technology.

Identify a champion in informatics or nursing leadership who is willing to pilot a tool. Try to conduct a small pilot with measurable outcomes: documentation time before and after, nurse satisfaction scores, error rates in documentation, etc. This data gives you the evidence you need to support a broader rollout. Offer to be part of the pilot team.

Connect to existing initiatives. Most healthcare organizations have active projects around nursing burnout, documentation burden, and staffing. AI documentation tools are a natural fit for all three. Find the project sponsor and make the connection explicit.

Case Study: The School Nurse Who Rebuilt Her Program

Keisha is a registered nurse and sole health provider for a K-8 school of 620 students. Her documentation requirements include health visit logs, medication administration records, care plans for students with chronic conditions, communication with parents, and annual health screenings. She has no administrative support and no other clinical staff. Before AI, much of her documentation happened after school hours or was deferred until it became urgent.

Her entry point was parent communication. She had a backlog of routine letters, follow-up notes after health visits, reminders about medication refills, and updates on students with chronic conditions that she could not get to during the school day. She started using a general AI tool for this purpose because none of her letters contained PHI. The results were immediate. Letters that took fifteen minutes each now took two to three minutes. She cleared her backlog in one week.

From there she built anonymized care plan templates for her most common student health conditions. Asthma, severe food allergies, type 1 diabetes, and seizure disorders. She used AI to generate comprehensive first drafts and then customized each one for the specific student. The quality of her care plans improved significantly because the AI-generated templates consistently included elements she might have abbreviated under time pressure.

Eighteen months in, Keisha describes her role differently. She spends less time on paperwork and more time with students. She has developed a training document for substitute nurses that she would not have had the time to create before. And she has started advocating within her district for a formal AI policy for school health services, using her own outcomes as evidence. Personal results are the most powerful argument for institutional support once you have them.

Case Study: The Oncology Unit That Built a Shared Library

The oncology unit at a regional cancer center had a documentation challenge specific to their patient population: chemotherapy education. Every patient starting a new regimen needed detailed individualized teaching about their specific drugs, their side effects, management strategies, and the warning signs that required an immediate call to the clinic. Each teaching session generated documentation that had to be thorough, accurate, and legally defensible. The nurses were doing this well, but it took significant time and the quality varied across the team.

The unit's clinical educator spent two weeks developing a set of chemotherapy education prompts, one for each of the twelve most common regimens used on the unit. Each prompt was specific to the regimen, included the correct drugs and their common side effects, it specified the reading level and format, and required the reviewing nurse to verify all clinical details against current pharmacy references before use.

The prompts were shared with the team via a simple shared document. Within a month, all twelve nurses on the unit were using them. Documentation time for chemotherapy teaching dropped by an estimated 40 percent. More significantly, quality became more consistent, every patient received a teaching document that covered the same essential elements, even when the nurse was new to that particular regimen.

Two outcomes surprised the team. First, newer nurses reported feeling more confident giving chemotherapy teaching because the structured prompt reminded them of elements they might have overlooked. Second, the shared prompt library became a living document. Nurses added notes when they found better language for a particular side effect or a more effective way to explain a management strategy. The AI tool became a platform for collective clinical knowledge. That outcome was not planned. It emerged from the practice.

What Nurses Can Do Right Now

The future of AI in nursing is being shaped now, not later. The nurses who understand these tools, use them thoughtfully, and can speak credibly about their implications are not passive observers of a technological shift. They are participants in it. Here is what that participation looks like in practical terms.

Use the tools and track your results. The most powerful evidence for AI adoption in any organization is a nurse who can say: before I integrated AI into my documentation workflow, I was charting for ninety minutes after every shift. Now I am done before I leave the unit. I have data. That nurse has more influence over institutional AI policy than any external vendor or consultant.

Engage with the governance structures at your facility. Most health systems are actively developing AI policies right now. If your organization has a nursing informatics committee, a technology governance board, or an AI task force, find out how to participate or submit input. The nursing perspective on how AI tools actually function at the bedside is systematically underrepresented in healthcare AI governance, and that gap has consequences for the tools that get approved and how they are implemented.

Stay connected to your professional organization. The ANA is actively developing guidance on AI in nursing practice. Specialty nursing organizations are doing the same. Staying current does not require hours of reading. Following one or two reliable nursing-focused publications and reviewing new ANA guidance when it is released is enough to keep your knowledge current without overwhelming your schedule.

Teach what you know. If you have built a working AI documentation practice, share it. Informal peer-to-peer teaching is how most clinical knowledge spreads in nursing. A demonstration during a break, a shared prompt, a five-minute conversation about what works. These small acts of knowledge sharing multiply across a unit and across a career. The nurses who will benefit most from AI tools are often the most skeptical, and the most effective messenger is a trusted colleague who has done it.

KEY TAKEAWAYS

- Nurses spend between 25 and 40 percent of their shift time on documentation, a burden that research consistently identifies as a primary driver of burnout and intent to leave the profession.
- AI is capable of helping with structured documentation drafting, patient education materials, shift handoff summaries, care planning support, and nurse self-reflection. It cannot assess patients, replace clinical judgment, guarantee accuracy, or accept accountability.
- The distinction between consumer AI tools and HIPAA-compliant healthcare AI tools is critical. **Consumer tools are not appropriate for clinical use.**
- The nurse retains full professional and ethical accountability for all AI-assisted documentation and decisions.

Chapter 2

Ethics, Scope of Practice, and Professional Accountability

The first question most nurses ask about AI is not how does it work. The first question is usually is it allowed. That is exactly the right question to ask first. Nursing is a licensed profession governed by a code of ethics, a scope of practice, and a regulatory framework that exists to protect patients. Before integrating any new tool into your clinical practice, understanding where that tool sits within those boundaries is not optional. It is a professional obligation.

The good news is that the nursing profession's governing bodies have done significant work to answer this question directly. The American Nurses Association updated its Code of Ethics in 2025 with specific language addressing AI. Its Ethics Advisory Board published a formal position statement on the ethical use of AI in nursing practice. The profession has taken a clear, considered, and practical position.

What the ANA Code of Ethics Actually Says:

The ANA Code of Ethics for Nurses was updated in 2025. Provision 4 is the most important for this conversation. It states that nurses have authority over nursing practice and are responsible and accountable for their practice. The interpretive statement accompanying Provision 4.2 is worth reading carefully: systems and technologies that assist in clinical practice are adjunct to, not replacements for, the nurse's knowledge and skill.

Adjunct to, not replacements for.

That phrase defines the entire framework for using AI in nursing. AI is a tool in your hands. The tool does not make decisions. You do. The tool does not hold a license. You do.

Provision 7.5, updated in 2025, addresses AI and machine learning specifically. It acknowledges that AI is already deeply embedded in healthcare and calls on nurses to stay informed about developments, acknowledge the potential benefits and harms, maintain the dignity of the patient, and ensure the voice of nursing is present in decisions about how technology is developed and applied. This is not a warning against using AI. It is a call to use it thoughtfully.

The ANA Position Statement on AI

In May 2025, the ANA Ethics Advisory Board published a formal position statement on the ethical use of AI in nursing practice. The core message is direct: the appropriate use of AI in nursing practice supports and enhances the core values and ethical obligations of the profession.

The position statement identifies four specific responsibilities for nurses who use AI tools:

1. Ensuring the validity of the AI tool being used
2. Ensuring the appropriate application of AI in the specific clinical context

3. Maintaining transparency in the process

4. Conducting ongoing evaluation for reliability

The statement also addresses accountability directly. Nurses who use AI to assist in documentation remain fully accountable for that documentation. The AI did not assess the patient. The AI did not make the clinical judgment. You did. Signing an AI-assisted note does not shift liability to the algorithm. It confirms that you, a licensed nurse, reviewed and approved the content as an accurate reflection of your clinical assessment and judgment.

The statement also emphasizes justice and equity as AI-specific concerns. AI systems can perpetuate and amplify biases present in the data they were trained on. A documentation tool trained predominantly on one patient population may produce outputs that are subtly inappropriate for another. Nurses, as patient advocates, have a responsibility to notice and raise concerns about inequitable AI performance.

Scope of Practice and the AI Boundary

AI integration does not change your scope of practice boundaries. What it changes is some of the work that happens within them.

Nursing assessment is within your scope. AI cannot conduct a nursing assessment. What AI can do is help you document an assessment you have already conducted, once you provide the clinical observations and findings. The boundary is clear. The assessment is yours. The documentation assistance is the tool's.

Clinical judgment is within your scope. AI cannot exercise clinical judgment. What AI can do is present information in a structured format, suggest note language based on patterns it has learned, or offer options for care plan language. You evaluate those suggestions using your clinical knowledge and judgment. You accept what is accurate and appropriate. You reject or modify what is not.

The boundary principle is consistent across every use case in this book: AI handles language and structure. Nursing handles assessment, judgment, and accountability. The moment you find yourself accepting AI output without genuinely reviewing it, or signing documentation that does not accurately reflect your clinical picture, you have crossed a line that your license and your patients cannot afford.

Core Ethical Principles Applied to AI

Beneficence means acting in the patient's best interest. AI-assisted documentation must accurately serve the patient's clinical needs. An efficiently produced but clinically inaccurate note does not serve the patient, regardless of how quickly it was generated.

Nonmaleficence means avoiding harm. AI can cause harm through inaccuracy, through bias, through uncritical acceptance of algorithmic output, and through exposure of patient information to non-compliant systems. Reviewing every AI output before it enters the clinical record is an act of nonmaleficence.

Autonomy means respecting the patient's right to make informed decisions. In the AI context, this includes being transparent with patients when AI tools are involved in their care documentation.

Justice means treating all patients equitably. Be alert to the possibility that AI tools perform differently for different patient populations and that AI-generated language may not appropriately reflect the diversity of patients in your care.

Fidelity means being faithful to your commitments as a nurse. Your commitment is that the documentation bearing your name accurately reflects the care you provided. AI can make documentation faster. Fidelity ensures it stays accurate.

The Accountability Standard

Before you sign any AI-assisted documentation, you are attesting that the content is accurate, that it reflects your clinical assessment and judgment, and that it meets the standards of your facility, your state's nursing practice act, and your professional code of ethics.

If that attestation is true, you have used AI appropriately. If it is not true, the AI did not cause the problem. The choice to accept inaccurate documentation caused the problem.

This distinction is not intended to create fear around AI use. It is intended to clarify where the professional responsibility sits, so that you can use AI with confidence when you use it correctly, and with appropriate caution when the temptation to cut corners arises.

KEY TAKEAWAYS

- The ANA 2025 Code of Ethics, Provision 4.2, is clear: systems and technologies that assist in clinical practice are adjunct to, not replacements for, the nurse's knowledge and skill.
- The ANA Position Statement on AI (2022, revised 2025) affirms that appropriate AI use supports and enhances the core values of nursing. Using AI well is consistent with ethical practice.
- Scope of practice boundaries do not change because AI is involved. Assessment, clinical judgment, and patient education are nursing functions. AI assists with language and structure.
- The five core ethical principles of nursing apply fully to AI-assisted practice and require active, thoughtful application at every step.
- The nurse who signs an AI-assisted note is fully accountable for its contents. Review every output. Correct what is wrong. Sign only what is accurate.

Chapter 3

HIPAA, Patient Privacy, and Data Security for Nurses

This is the chapter that determines whether you use AI safely or not. Everything else in this book depends on getting this right. You can write the best prompts in the world, but if you are sending them to a tool that is not HIPAA compliant, you are creating a liability every single time you use it.

What HIPAA Means for AI Use

HIPAA, the Health Insurance Portability and Accountability Act, governs how Protected Health Information is used, stored, and transmitted. PHI is any information that could be used to identify a specific patient in connection with their health status, healthcare services, or payment for care. A patient's name is PHI. A date of birth is PHI. A room number, a diagnosis, a medication list, an account number, all PHI.

The rule that matters most for AI use: PHI cannot be shared with a third party without either the patient's authorization or a signed Business Associate Agreement between your organization and that third party. When you type information about a patient into any AI tool, you are transmitting data to that tool's servers. The question is whether that tool has a BAA with your organization.

Why Consumer AI Tools Are Not Appropriate for Clinical Use

The free version of ChatGPT, the standard consumer version of Claude, the general-purpose Gemini interface, none of these have signed BAAs with your hospital, your clinic, or your home health agency. They were not designed for healthcare use. When you type patient information into one of these tools, that data may be used to train future AI models, may be stored on servers that do not meet healthcare security standards, and is outside the protection of any healthcare compliance framework.

This does not mean these tools are bad. It means they were built for a different purpose. There is one important exception: if you are using these general AI tools for tasks that involve absolutely zero patient information such as drafting a professional development reflection, generating ideas for an in-service training, writing a care plan template without any patient data, the HIPAA concern does not apply.

What Makes a Tool HIPAA Compliant

For a tool to be used safely with patient-related content:

- The vendor must be willing to sign a Business Associate Agreement
- The tool must use encryption in transit and at rest
- The tool must have a clear data retention and deletion policy
- The tool must meet the technical safeguards of the HIPAA Security Rule

When evaluating a tool, the fastest first step is to ask your compliance or informatics team whether the tool has been approved for clinical use at your facility.

Tools Available in 2026

Healthcare-Specific Ambient Documentation

Purpose-built platforms such as Nuance DAX Express and Suki are designed to process clinical input through HIPAA-compliant systems and generate structured documentation. These tools generally have BAAs available and are designed for institutional use. Nursing-specific versions are in development and some are already deployed.

EHR-Integrated AI Features

Epic and similar EHR systems are rolling out AI documentation assistance features within their platforms. Since these features exist within your facility's existing infrastructure, they inherit the compliance protections already in place. If your EHR has AI features available for nursing documentation, these are worth exploring first.

Enterprise Versions of General AI Tools

Microsoft Azure OpenAI and Google Cloud AI services can be configured to meet HIPAA requirements, including BAA signing. If your facility has an enterprise agreement that includes AI services, those tools may be compliant for clinical use. Check with your compliance team before assuming.

The Anonymization Approach

Here is a practical middle ground that many nurses use when working with a general AI tool: remove all PHI before composing your prompt. Use clinical descriptors only.

Acceptable: A 67-year-old male with a history of heart failure admitted for worsening shortness of breath.
Not acceptable: John Smith in room 412 with CHF.

This approach lets you use general AI tools for the structural and language work without transmitting protected information. You draft the anonymized prompt, receive the structured output, then fill in accurate patient-specific details when you enter documentation into your facility's EHR. This is not a substitute for using a properly compliant tool. It is a practical option for specific tasks where no patient data needs to be involved in the AI interaction at all.

Practical Rules for Daily Use

- Never enter a patient's name into a consumer AI tool, not even a first name in combination with any clinical information
- Never enter a patient's date of birth, medical record number, room number, or any number that could identify them
- Never copy and paste directly from your EHR into a consumer AI tool without first removing all identifying information
- If your facility has approved specific tools for clinical AI use, use those
- Always keep final documentation in your EHR, where it belongs

KEY TAKEAWAYS

- PHI is any information that could identify a patient in connection with their health. Any combination of name, date, room number, or identifier with clinical information is PHI and must be handled accordingly.
- Consumer AI tools in their standard form do not have Business Associate Agreements with healthcare organizations and are not appropriate for use with patient-identifiable information.
- For a tool to be used safely with PHI, it must have a signed BAA, use appropriate encryption, have a clear data policy, and meet HIPAA Security Rule requirements.
- EHR-integrated AI features and healthcare-specific platforms are the safest options because their compliance frameworks are already established.
- The anonymization approach lets you use general tools for structural drafting tasks when no patient-specific information needs to be involved.

Chapter 4

Prompt Engineering Basics for Nurses

You do not need to be a programmer or a technology expert to write a good prompt. Prompt engineering is just the skill of communicating clearly with an AI tool so that you get useful output instead of generic, vague, or wrong output.

Think of it this way. If you handed a new nursing assistant a piece of paper and said write me a note, you would get something. But if you said write me a one-paragraph summary of this patient's status, using SBAR format, focusing on the respiratory assessment and the medication changes from today's shift, you would get something much more useful. Prompting AI works the same way.

The Five Elements of a Nursing Prompt

Every effective nursing prompt contains some combination of five elements. You do not always need all five, but knowing each one helps you build prompts that work.

Role tells the AI what perspective to take. Saying Act as a registered nurse or You are an experienced ICU nurse helps the AI calibrate its language and the appropriate level of clinical detail. Without a role, the AI defaults to a generalist perspective that may not match clinical standards.

Task tells the AI what you want it to produce. Be specific. Prompting AI to write a DAR note is better than just prompting it to write a note. The task description is the most important element of your prompt!

Context gives the AI the information it needs to produce accurate output. This is where you include your anonymized clinical details, the patient's relevant history, the interventions you performed, and the patient's response. More relevant context produces more accurate output.

Format tells the AI how to structure the output. Do you want SBAR, DAR, SOAP, PIE, or a different format? Do you want bullet points or paragraphs? A specific word count? Specifying format saves editing time.

Constraints tell the AI what to avoid. Do not include any diagnostic conclusions or keep this under 150 words are constraints that improve output quality and safety.

Basic Prompt Examples

Shift Handoff Summary

> **PROMPT:** You are a registered nurse preparing an end-of-shift SBAR handoff. Using the following anonymized patient data, write a clear SBAR summary that the incoming nurse can use to take over care. Keep it under 200 words. Do not include any diagnostic conclusions. [Patient data here]

Patient Education Handout

> **PROMPT:** You are a registered nurse creating patient education materials. Write a simple, plain-language handout explaining how to care for a surgical wound at home. Use a 6th grade reading level. Include when to call the doctor. Format it with short paragraphs and a brief bullet list of warning signs.

Care Plan Goal

> **PROMPT:** You are a registered nurse writing a nursing care plan. Create three SMART goals for a patient with decreased mobility following hip replacement surgery. Each goal should be measurable within a 48-hour timeframe and should address a different aspect of recovery: pain, mobility, and fall prevention.

Intermediate Techniques

Once you are comfortable with basic prompts, a few intermediate techniques will improve your results significantly.

Give an example. If you have a well-written DAR note from a previous shift, you can include it as a model and say write a similar note using this format and this level of detail. AI is good at pattern matching, and an example is often more effective than a long description of what you want.

Ask for step-by-step reasoning. For more complex tasks, adding "think through this step by step" to your prompt often produces more accurate and complete output. This is particularly useful for care planning and clinical reasoning tasks.

Ask the AI to flag its gaps. Adding a line like flag any areas where you need more information to complete this accurately produces output that tells you where you need to add clinical detail. This is a useful quality check.

Use follow-up prompts. You do not have to get everything right in your first prompt. If the output is almost right but needs adjustment, tell the AI what to change: make this shorter, use simpler language, add a section on activity restrictions.

Common Mistakes and How to Fix Them

The most common mistake is asking for too much in one prompt. If you need a SOAP note, three patient education materials, and a care plan, break those into separate prompts. Complex multi-part requests produce inconsistent results.

The second most common mistake is forgetting to specify the audience. A prompt that does not specify whether the output is for a clinical colleague, a patient, or a family member will produce something that may be appropriate for none of them. Always say who the output is for.

The third mistake is accepting the first output without reading it carefully. AI produces plausible-sounding language quickly. Plausible-sounding is not the same as clinically accurate. Read every output before you use it.

KEY TAKEAWAYS

- Prompt engineering is the skill of giving AI clear, specific instructions that produce useful output. It does not require technical expertise, just clarity about what you want.
- Every effective nursing prompt contains some combination of five elements: role, task, context, format, and constraints. The more specific your prompt, the better your output.
- Intermediate techniques include giving examples of good output, asking AI to think step by step, asking it to flag its own gaps, and using follow-up prompts to refine results.
- Common mistakes are asking for too much in one prompt, forgetting to specify the audience, and accepting output without reading it carefully.

Chapter 5

Building Safe, Effective Prompts for Clinical Use

Chapter 4 taught you the structure of a good prompt. This chapter adds the safety layer that makes prompts appropriate for clinical nursing contexts. Nursing prompts are different from general AI prompts because the stakes are different. An AI-generated nursing note that is slightly off and goes into a patient record without review can harm a patient or expose you to liability. The seven principles in this chapter are specifically designed to prevent that.

Principle 1: Define the Role and Its Limits

Every nursing prompt should establish both what the AI is and what it is not. Defining the role as registered nurse or nursing documentation assistant sets the appropriate clinical register. Adding a limiting statement sets a boundary that shapes all subsequent output.

EXAMPLE: You are a registered nurse assisting with documentation. You organize and structure clinical information provided by the nurse. You do not assess patients, make diagnostic conclusions, or suggest clinical interventions unless asked to generate options for the nurse to review.

Principle 2: Mandate Anonymization and Zero PHI

Build the anonymization requirement directly into every prompt for clinical documentation tasks:

INCLUDE: Do not include any patient name, date of birth, room number, medical record number, or any other identifying information in your output. Use clinical descriptors only.

Principle 3: Stay Evidence-Based

Clinical content in AI output should be grounded in standard nursing practice. For care planning or patient education prompts, include a requirement that grounds AI output in current nursing standards:

INCLUDE: Base all clinical recommendations on evidence-based nursing practice. Do not include interventions or information that is not consistent with current nursing standards.

Principle 4: Require Step-by-Step Reasoning for Complex Tasks

For prompts that involve clinical reasoning tasks like care planning, asking the AI to show its reasoning helps you catch errors before they reach the final product. This produces output that is easier to evaluate because you can see the logic, not just the conclusion.

INCLUDE: Think through this step by step, showing your reasoning before presenting the final output.

Principle 5: Specify Output Format Precisely

Vague format instructions produce variable output. Precise format instructions produce consistent output that requires less editing.

EXAMPLE: Write a DAR note with three clearly labeled sections: Data, Action, Response. Each section should be one to three sentences. Use past tense. Use objective clinical language.

Principle 6: Require Human Review Reminders

Build a human review reminder directly into every clinical documentation prompt. This keeps the review step visible and intentional, and documents that oversight was built into your process.

INCLUDE: End your output with this reminder: [REQUIRES NURSE REVIEW AND CLINICAL VERIFICATION BEFORE USE]

Principle 7: Maintain a Personal Prompt Library

Your prompts will improve over time. Keep a personal prompt library where you save and date your prompt templates. When you update a prompt because you found a better way to structure it, keep the previous version so you can compare results. A prompt library is covered in full in Appendix A, and Chapter 6 shows you how to use it.

The Master Prompt Template

Combining all seven principles, here is the master template that underlies every nursing prompt in the Appendix A library:

MASTER TEMPLATE: You are a registered nurse assisting with documentation. You organize and structure clinical information provided by the nurse. You do not assess patients, make diagnostic conclusions, or suggest clinical interventions beyond presenting options for the nurse to review. Do not include any patient name, date of birth, room number, or any other identifying information in your output. Base all clinical content on evidence-based nursing practice standards. [TASK DESCRIPTION]. [CLINICAL CONTEXT, ANONYMIZED]. [FORMAT SPECIFICATION]. [CONSTRAINTS IF ANY]. End your output with: [REQUIRES NURSE REVIEW AND CLINICAL VERIFICATION BEFORE USE]

Putting the Template Into Practice

The master template above is not meant to be copied word for word every single time. It is meant to become internalized so that the safety elements become automatic habits rather than a checklist you consult. Most nurses who have been using clinical AI prompts for two or three months report that they no longer think about the seven principles individually. They have become the way they construct prompts naturally.

The fastest path to that internalization is repetition on low-stakes tasks. Before you use the master template on a real clinical note, use it five times on fictional scenarios. Notice what each element does to the output quality. Notice what happens when you leave one out. The learning curve is short. Most nurses reach confident fluency within two to three weeks of consistent daily use.

One practical adaptation that many nurses find useful is keeping a shortened version of the master template as a saved note on their phone. The full template runs about 80 words. A shortened version that includes role, anonymization reminder, task, format, and review reminder is enough to produce quality output once the habits are established. Start with the full version. Condense as you build fluency.

Quick Pre-Submission Checklist

Before submitting any clinical prompt, run through these questions. It takes about five seconds once you have done it a few times:

- Have I defined the role and its limits?
- Have I removed all PHI from my input?
- Have I specified the output format?
- Have I included a constraint that matches my clinical context?
- Does this prompt ask AI to do only what a documentation tool should do?
- Have I included the human review reminder?

KEY TAKEAWAYS

- The seven principles of safe clinical prompting are: define the role and its limits, mandate anonymization, require evidence-based content, ask for step-by-step reasoning on complex tasks, specify output format precisely, require human review reminders, and maintain version control of your prompts.
- The master prompt template combines all seven principles into a reusable structure. Every prompt in the Appendix A library is built on this template.
- The human review reminder should appear at the end of every clinical documentation output as a visible, consistent practice.

Chapter 6
Working With the Nursing Prompt Library

How the Six Categories Map to Your Workday

Appendix A contains 60 prompts organized into six categories. This chapter is your guide to using them. The prompts were designed using the seven principles from Chapter 5. They are ready to use, but they are not finished products. Every prompt is a starting point that you customize with your specific clinical context.

Category 1 covers Shift Preparation and Handoff Documentation: reviewing patient summaries, prioritizing care order, preparing handoff reports, and documenting the transfer of care.

Category 2 covers Clinical Notes and Charting: SOAP, DAR, PIE, and Focus Charting formats. This is the category most nurses reach for first.

Category 3 covers Care Planning and Goal Setting: nursing care plans, SMART goals, and care conferences.

Category 4 covers Patient Education Materials: plain-language handouts, discharge instructions, medication teaching aids, and procedure explanations.

Category 5 covers Between-Shift and Administrative Support: policy lookups, competency documentation, email drafting, and professional development reflections.

Category 6 covers Nurse Self-Care and Reflection: post-shift debriefs, stress processing, and professional boundary-setting support. These prompts are for you, not for the chart.

Three Principles Before You Begin

The prompt is a tool, not a substitute for assessment. Every prompt in this library asks you for clinical context as input. That context comes from your assessment. The quality of what you put in determines the quality of what comes out. Vague input produces vague output.

The output is a draft, not a final document. Every output from every prompt requires your review. Read it completely. Add what is missing. Correct what is wrong. Remove what does not apply. Then and only then does it become documentation.

Your judgment is the final filter. If the output does not match your clinical picture, trust your clinical judgment over the AI output. The AI does not know your patient. You do.

Building Your Personal Prompt Library

The 60 prompts in Appendix A are the starting point, not the whole library. Over time, you will modify prompts to fit your specific unit, your specific EHR format, your specific patient population, and your own clinical voice. When you modify a prompt and get better results, save the new version. Name it clearly. Date it.

Your personal prompt library is a professional asset. It represents your clinical experience translated into a structured tool. It travels with you if you change units or facilities. And it gets better with every shift you work.

KEY TAKEAWAYS

- The six prompt categories map directly to the main areas of nursing documentation time: shift prep and handoff, clinical notes, care planning, patient education, administrative support, and self-care.
- Three principles apply before using any prompt: the prompt is a tool not a substitute for assessment, the output is a draft not a final document, and your clinical judgment is the final filter.
- The highest-use category for most nurses is clinical notes. The most important habit is reading every output carefully before approving it.
- Building a personal prompt library over time is a professional development practice. Modified and refined prompts that fit your specific clinical context are more valuable than generic starting templates.

Chapter 7

AI-Assisted Shift Preparation and Patient Handoff

Why These Tasks Are Well-Suited for AI

If there is one area where nurses consistently report the fastest and most tangible benefit from AI, it is shift prep and handoff. Shift prep and handoff documentation share a characteristic that makes them ideal for AI assistance: they are largely about organizing and structuring information you already have, not generating new clinical content. That conversion is exactly what AI is good at.

The beginning of a shift is often chaotic. You are receiving a verbal handoff from a tired nurse, scanning through chart entries from the past several hours, checking on pending orders, reviewing vitals trends, and trying to build a mental model of four to eight patients in fifteen minutes. The end of a shift is similar: you are exhausted and have to organize everything you did for the past twelve hours into something coherent for the nurse who is about to take over.

The SBAR Framework and AI

SBAR stands for Situation, Background, Assessment, and Recommendation. It is one of the most widely used structured communication frameworks in nursing and healthcare. It is also a format that AI handles very well because it has a clear, consistent structure with defined content for each section.

When you give AI anonymized clinical information and ask it to structure that information into SBAR format, the output is usually well-organized and complete. Your job is to review it for clinical accuracy and add the qualitative observations that do not come from data alone: the patient who seems more anxious than usual, the family dynamic affecting care, the small vital trend that is not alarming yet but that you have been watching.

Core Shift Prep Workflow

As you receive your verbal handoff and scan the chart, take brief notes using anonymized identifiers and clinical descriptors rather than names. Once you have notes on all patients, open your shift prep prompt, paste in your anonymized notes, and submit. Review the output for clinical accuracy and add qualitative observations from your bedside assessment. Use the output as your working reference for the shift, not as a replacement for ongoing assessment.

For end-of-shift handoff: in the last hour of your shift, collect your shift documentation for each patient. Anonymize it. Open your SBAR handoff prompt. For each patient, input the key information: what was their status at start of shift, what significant events or changes occurred, what interventions were performed and how the patient responded, what is outstanding, and anything specific the incoming nurse needs to know.

AI-generated handoff summaries consistently miss the qualitative observations that come from being at the bedside. The nurse's role in reviewing and supplementing the output with this information is not optional. It is the clinical value-add that makes the handoff safe.

KEY TAKEAWAYS

- Shift prep and handoff are well-suited for AI assistance because they involve organizing information you already have, not generating new clinical content.
- SBAR is a natural fit for AI-assisted handoff because its clear four-section structure produces consistent, well-organized output when combined with good anonymized clinical input.
- The core workflow is: collect anonymized notes during the shift, submit to your handoff prompt, review and add qualitative observations, and use the result for verbal and written handoff.
- AI-generated handoffs consistently miss the qualitative observations that come from being at the bedside. Adding this information is not optional.

Chapter 8

AI-Assisted Clinical Documentation and Charting

Note Formats Covered in This Chapter

This is the chapter most nurses turn to first, and for good reason. Documentation is where the hours go. The average nurse spends between 25 and 40 percent of a shift in front of a screen, converting clinical observations into written records. A significant portion of that time is structural: choosing words, formatting sections, organizing data into the right template. That portion is where AI adds real value.

SOAP notes organize documentation into four sections: Subjective (what the patient reports), Objective (measurable clinical data), Assessment (the nurse's interpretation), and Plan (the nursing plan of care going forward). SOAP is widely used across settings.

DAR notes stand for Data, Action, and Response, organized around what the nurse observed or assessed, what the nurse did, and how the patient responded. DAR is common in long-term care, behavioral health, and home health settings.

PIE notes organize documentation into Problem, Intervention, and Evaluation sections. PIE is used in some acute care settings and is particularly useful for documenting specific nursing problems and the interventions addressing them.

Focus Charting uses a DAR structure centered on a specific focus, a symptom, a condition, a patient concern, or a nursing diagnosis rather than a comprehensive shift summary.

Core Documentation Workflow With AI

Conduct your assessment at the bedside. This is the clinical work that AI cannot do. Your observations, your physical assessment findings, your clinical judgment about what you are seeing. All of that happens before AI enters the picture.

Collect your data in brief, anonymized notes. A list of bullet points with your objective findings, a brief note about the subjective report, your assessment of the situation, and the interventions you performed is enough.

Open your documentation prompt, specify the format, paste in your anonymized clinical data, and submit. Read the output from beginning to end. Verify every clinical statement. Correct errors. Add missing detail. Remove anything that does not apply to this patient's situation. Then copy the reviewed and corrected output into your EHR.

Common Documentation Errors AI Makes

AI sometimes fills gaps with assumptions. If your input is incomplete, the AI may generate plausible-sounding content to fill the empty space rather than leaving it blank or flagging it as missing. Always include the instruction "do not add clinical information not present in the input".

AI sometimes uses imprecise language that sounds clinical but lacks specificity. If you read "patient appears comfortable" without any supporting data, that is an unspecific statement. Catch these phrases and replace them with specific observations.

AI sometimes misinterprets clinical shorthand. If your notes use abbreviations that have multiple meanings in different contexts, the AI may interpret them incorrectly. When in doubt, spell it out in your prompt input.

AI sometimes combines information from multiple patients if your input accidentally includes data from more than one. Double-check your input before submitting.

Documentation Timing: During the Shift vs. After

One of the most important workflow decisions for AI-assisted documentation is timing. Most nurses default to end-of-shift charting because that is the established habit. AI-assisted documentation works significantly better when the cognitive work happens during the shift rather than after it.

The practical approach: carry a notes app on your phone or badge reel during the shift. After each significant patient interaction, an assessment, an intervention, a family conversation, a change in condition, take sixty seconds to dictate a brief, anonymized summary of what happened and what you did. These micro-notes take almost no time at the moment and are infinitely better than trying to reconstruct twelve hours from memory at 8 PM.

At the end of your shift, you are not trying to remember. You are organizing. Open your documentation prompt, paste in the micro-notes for each patient in turn, and let AI do the structural work. The review takes minutes rather than hours because you are verifying, not reconstructing.

This shift from after-the-fact documentation to continuous micro-documentation is the single biggest workflow change that nurses report making once they are comfortable with AI tools. It feels counterintuitive at first. It feels like one more thing to do during an already busy shift. Within two to three weeks it becomes automatic, and the end of the shift feels completely different.

Case Vignette: From Two Hours to Twenty Minutes

Theresa is a med-surg nurse with twelve years of experience. Before AI, her end-of-shift charting routine took between ninety minutes and two hours for a four-patient assignment. Now she dictates brief anonymized summaries for each patient during the last two hours of her shift while she is still actively working. At shift end, she spends about five minutes submitting those notes to her documentation prompts and reviewing the output. The actual charting takes about twenty minutes for four patients.

What changed was not the quality of her documentation. It is, if anything, more thorough than before, because the structured format consistently reminds her to include sections she might have rushed through at the end of a long shift. What changed was where the cognitive work happens: during the shift, while she is with her patients, rather than after the shift when she is exhausted.

The time she reclaimed is not just time. It is the difference between getting home at a reasonable hour and sitting in the parking lot at midnight too tired to drive safely. She reports that she thinks she is a better nurse because she is less depleted. AI did not change her clinical skills. It changed what she had left over after using them.

KEY TAKEAWAYS

- SOAP, DAR, PIE, and Focus Charting are the four most common nursing documentation formats. AI handles all of them effectively when given a clear format specification and accurate anonymized clinical input.
- The core documentation workflow is: assess at the bedside, collect anonymized notes, submit to your documentation prompt, review the output completely, correct errors, enter into EHR.
- AI makes four common documentation errors: filling gaps with assumptions, using imprecise language, misinterpreting clinical shorthand, and combining information from multiple patients.
- The time savings from AI documentation are most significant at the end of shifts when fatigue is highest and documentation quality is most at risk.

Chapter 9
Patient Education Materials and Care Instructions

Why AI Excels at Patient Education Drafting

Creating patient education materials is one of the most time-consuming tasks in nursing that also has one of the clearest AI use cases. AI can do most of the structural and language work in under a minute, leaving you to verify clinical accuracy and customize for the specific patient.

Patient education materials follow predictable structures. A medication teaching handout has recognizable sections: what this medication is, how to take it, what side effects to watch for, and when to call your provider. AI is good at generating content within established structures.

They need to be written at a specific reading level. Most patient education materials should be written at a sixth to eighth grade reading level. AI, when instructed, produces readable plain-language content more consistently than most humans writing under time pressure.

They often do not contain PHI by default. Patient education materials are typically generic clinical content rather than patient-specific documentation. This means they can often be drafted using general AI tools even at facilities without HIPAA-compliant clinical AI, as long as you are generating generic content that you then customize.

Clear Boundaries for AI in Patient Education

AI should not be the final clinical authority on any care instruction. Medication dosing information, procedural care steps, and activity restrictions should be verified against your facility's approved materials, the patient's specific orders, and current evidence-based practice before being given to a patient.

AI should not replace your facility's standard approved education materials where they exist. AI is most valuable when no approved standard material exists, when you need to customize a standard piece significantly for a specific patient, or when you need to create something quickly in a situation where no standard exists.

AI should not produce education materials in languages you cannot verify for accuracy. Machine translation errors in patient education can be serious. If a patient needs materials in a language other than English, the AI translation should be reviewed by a qualified interpreter before being given to the patient.

Reading Level, Language, and Health Literacy

Reading level matters more than nurses often realize. The average American adult reads at approximately an eighth grade level, and many patients read at a lower level. Specify the reading level in every patient education prompt. Sixth grade is a safe default for general patient populations.

Language access is a patient rights issue, not a courtesy. Patients with limited English proficiency have a right to materials in a language they can understand. AI can produce reasonable first-draft translations that are useful as a starting point. They require review by a qualified interpreter before being given to a patient.

Health literacy encompasses not just reading ability but the capacity to understand and act on health information. Short sentences, active voice, specific action-oriented language, and visual organization all improve health literacy access. AI, when prompted correctly, produces content with these features.

KEY TAKEAWAYS

- Patient education materials are well-suited for AI drafting because they follow predictable structures, benefit from plain-language writing, require completeness, and often do not contain PHI.

- AI output for patient education requires clinical verification before being given to a patient. Every specific clinical recommendation should be checked against current orders and evidence-based practice.

- Use your facility's approved standard materials when they exist. AI is most valuable when no standard material exists, when significant customization is needed, or when you need to create something quickly.

- Specify reading level in every patient education prompt. Sixth grade is a reliable default. Verify any AI translation with a qualified interpreter before giving it to a patient.

Chapter 10
Specialty Nursing Workflows

ICU and Critical Care

Critical care nurses document constantly. Hourly assessments, hemodynamic values, ventilator settings, vasoactive drip adjustments, fluid balance calculations, and multisystem status updates create a documentation volume that is among the highest in nursing practice.

Where AI helps most in critical care is synthesis work. You have all the data. Turning it into a coherent shift narrative takes time. AI can draft the structure of that narrative from your anonymized inputs quickly.

Where to be careful: the complexity of critical care patients means that AI errors in documentation carry higher stakes than in lower-acuity settings. A note that incorrectly characterizes a hemodynamic trend or misrepresents a medication adjustment in a critically ill patient can have consequences for care coordination. Review with extra attention in this setting.

Emergency Department

ED nursing documentation has its own particular challenge: speed. AI is most useful in the ED for triage documentation, SBAR handoffs for admission or transfer, and patient education materials for discharge instructions.

Where to be careful: the pace of the emergency department means the temptation to accept AI output without thorough review is higher than in other settings. Build in the habit of a thirty-second review minimum for any AI-generated content before it goes into a chart, even in a busy ED.

Pediatric Nursing

When writing family education materials for a pediatric patient, specify in your prompt that the audience is the parent or caregiver, not the patient. Specify the child's age range because the vocabulary and complexity of the explanation should reflect what is appropriate for a caregiver.

Pediatric weight-based medication dosing, developmental considerations in care planning, and age-specific normal ranges for vital signs are all areas where AI may produce content based on adult norms. Flag these areas explicitly in your prompts and verify any pediatric-specific values against current references.

Behavioral Health Nursing

Behavioral health nursing uses documentation formats that emphasize mental status, behavioral observations, and therapeutic interventions differently than medical-surgical nursing. DAR and PIE formats are common. Mental status examination documentation has specific elements that need to be present for clinical and legal purposes.

Documentation in this setting often has more significant legal implications than in other settings. Involuntary holds, competency evaluations, and safety risk documentation all require particular precision. AI should be used with heightened review standards for any behavioral health documentation that may have legal implications.

Home Health and Community Nursing

Home health nurses face a documentation challenge that is somewhat the reverse of hospital nurses: they often do most of their documentation at home, away from the clinical environment, working from notes taken in the field. AI is valuable in home health for OASIS documentation assistance, visit note structuring, and care plan updates.

The HIPAA considerations are particularly important for home health nurses who use personal devices for documentation. Make sure any AI tool you use meets compliance requirements and that your agency has approved it for clinical use.

Nurse Practitioners and Advanced Practice Roles

Nurse practitioners and other advanced practice nurses have a documentation burden that combines the nursing documentation requirements of their clinical role with the provider-level requirements of their prescribing and diagnostic authority. SOAP notes for NP encounters need to include differential thinking, a physical examination section, and a plan that addresses diagnosis, medication management, referrals, and follow-up.

AI handles NP-level documentation well when the prompt specifies the advanced practice context. Be explicit in your prompt that the role is a nurse practitioner completing a full visit note, specify the format requirements of your practice, and include the clinical context for the patient encounter.

KEY TAKEAWAYS

- Critical care AI documentation is most useful for shift narrative synthesis but requires especially careful review given the complexity and stakes of critical care patient documentation.
- ED nursing AI is most useful for triage documentation and discharge education but requires a disciplined review habit given the time pressure in emergency settings.
- Pediatric documentation prompts need to explicitly specify pediatric context, and pediatric-specific values require verification against current references.
- Behavioral health documentation with legal implications should receive heightened review standards.
- Home health nurses should ensure their AI tools are approved for clinical use given the HIPAA considerations of personal device use in field documentation.

Chapter 11
Comparing AI Tools for Nurses in 2026

Evaluation Criteria

Not all AI tools are equal, and the differences are not just about features. They are about compliance, data handling, output quality, and fit for clinical use.

HIPAA compliance comes first. Does the vendor offer a Business Associate Agreement? Has your facility approved the tool? If the answer to either question is no, the tool is not appropriate for any documentation that involves patient information. This is not negotiable.

Data retention and model training policy matters significantly. What happens to your inputs after you submit them? Does the vendor use your prompts and outputs to train their AI models? For clinical content, you want a vendor who does not use your data for training and who has a clear data deletion policy.

Healthcare-specific design matters. Was the tool built for healthcare use or adapted from a general-purpose AI? Tools built specifically for clinical documentation generally produce more accurate clinical language and are less likely to generate plausible-but-wrong clinical content.

Integration with your EHR reduces friction and the risk of transcription errors. EHR-integrated AI is the gold standard for documentation assistance. Ease of use on a busy shift is also a practical criterion: a tool that requires fifteen steps to generate a note will not be used consistently.

Categories of Tools in 2026

Healthcare-specific ambient documentation platforms are the premium option for clinical AI. Tools like Nuance DAX Express are designed for clinical input and produce structured documentation that integrates with the EHR. Nursing-specific versions of these platforms are actively being developed and deployed.

EHR-integrated AI features are emerging rapidly. Epic has been developing and deploying AI documentation assistance features within the platform. Because these features exist within your facility's existing EHR infrastructure, they inherit the compliance frameworks already in place.

Enterprise AI platforms are the compliant versions of general AI tools. Microsoft Azure OpenAI and Google Cloud AI services can be configured for HIPAA compliance and may be available to nurses through enterprise agreements that your facility has with these vendors.

Consumer AI tools with HIPAA add-ons: some vendors offer HIPAA-compliant tiers of otherwise consumer-facing tools. ChatGPT Enterprise, for example, includes HIPAA compliance options and does not use customer data for model training. These options require institutional agreements and are not the same as the free consumer version.

The Hybrid Approach

Most experienced nurses who have integrated AI into their practice use more than one tool. A common pattern is to use their facility's approved clinical tool for patient-adjacent documentation and a general AI tool for the non-clinical administrative and professional development tasks where HIPAA is not a concern.

A simple personal rule that works: if the task involves a specific patient or specific patient data, it goes to the compliant tool. Everything else can go to a general tool. Keeping the boundary clear between clinical and non-clinical AI use is the key to making this approach work safely.

KEY TAKEAWAYS

- HIPAA compliance and BAA availability are the non-negotiable first criteria for any tool used with patient information.
- Healthcare-specific ambient documentation tools and EHR-integrated AI features are the safest options because their compliance frameworks are purpose-built for clinical use.
- Enterprise versions of consumer AI tools can be configured for HIPAA compliance but require institutional agreements.
- Most experienced nurses use a hybrid approach: a compliant tool for patient-adjacent tasks and a general tool for non-clinical professional tasks.

Chapter 12

Step-by-Step Implementation for Nurses

Before You Begin

Reading about AI is different from using it. This chapter gives you the specific steps to go from reading this book to actively using AI in your nursing practice in a way that is safe, confident, and sustainable. The plan is organized into four phases spread across about ten weeks.

Two things need to happen before you start. First, find out what your facility has approved. Talk to your charge nurse, your nurse manager, or your informatics team. Ask specifically whether the facility has approved any AI documentation tools and whether there are policies governing personal AI use for clinical tasks.

Second, set up one compliant tool. If your facility has an approved tool, set up your access. If your facility does not have an approved tool and you are going to use the anonymization approach with a general AI tool, choose one that you will use consistently. Consistency builds skill faster than using different tools randomly.

Phase 1: Preparation (Weeks 1 to 2)

In the first two weeks, your only goal is to get familiar with how the tool works before you use it for anything that touches patient care. Spend fifteen minutes experimenting with prompts that have no clinical stakes. Ask the AI to write a professional bio for a fictional nurse. Ask it to explain the SBAR format as if teaching a new graduate. Ask it to draft a polite email declining a committee assignment.

Notice how the quality of output changes when you change your prompts. Add a role and see if the output improves. Add a format instruction. Add a constraint. The principles from Chapters 4 and 5 become intuitive much faster when you practice them on low-stakes tasks.

Phase 2: Safe Experimentation (Weeks 3 to 6)

Start with patient education materials only. Choose a commonly used education topic in your specialty. Use your prompt library to draft a patient education handout on that topic with no patient-specific information in the prompt. Review the output, compare it to your standard materials, and assess the quality and accuracy.

Once you are comfortable with education materials, move to handoff preparation. At the end of one shift, draft an anonymized prompt from your patient notes and generate a handoff summary. Compare it to your standard handoff. Is it more or less complete? What did you have to add or correct?

Keep a brief log of what works and what needs adjustment. Even a few notes in your phone about this type of prompt works well or this output always needs this correction is enough to accelerate your learning.

Phase 3: Building Habits (Weeks 7 to 10)

In weeks 7 through 10, AI becomes part of your regular workflow rather than something you try occasionally. Establish one specific point in your shift where you consistently use AI. For most nurses, this is either the last hour of the shift for documentation, or a specific point early in the shift for preparation and prioritization.

Begin building your personal prompt library. Take the prompts from Appendix A that you have been using and modify them to fit your specific documentation format, your specific patient population, and your own clinical voice.

Phase 4: Full Integration and Long-Term Sustainability

By week 10 and beyond, AI should feel like a normal part of how you practice. The markers of successful integration: your documentation quality is at least as high as it was before, your end-of-shift charting time has decreased measurably, and you no longer have to consciously remember to use the tool, it is just part of how you work.

Long-term sustainability requires two ongoing practices. The first is continuing to update your prompt library as you find better approaches and as your clinical context evolves. The second is staying informed about tool updates, policy changes, and new options as the AI landscape continues to evolve. Your facility's informatics team and the ANA's ongoing guidance are both good sources for this.

One marker that separates sustained adopters from those who eventually drift back to old habits: the nurses who sustain AI integration are the ones who have connected the time savings to something they genuinely value. More sleep. More time with family. The ability to exercise after a shift rather than collapse. Keep that connection visible. When you are tired and tempted to skip the prompt and just chart from scratch, remembering what you are protecting makes the difference.

Bringing Your Team Along

If you are a solo nurse reading this book, your adoption path is straightforward: you decide to use the tools and you build the habit. If you are a charge nurse, clinical educator, or nurse manager, you have an opportunity to accelerate adoption across your team that is worth thinking about deliberately.

The most common mistake in team AI adoption is mandating use before demonstrating value. People do not change how they work because they are told to. They change when they see something clearly making their job easier. The more effective approach: build the habit yourself over Phase 1 and 2, identify the two or three workflows where AI consistently saves you significant time, and then show those specific workflows to one or two colleagues. Walk them through the prompt, show them the output, and let them see how much time it saves.

Peer-to-peer demonstration is the most effective adoption mechanism in clinical settings. A nurse who sees another nurse leave the unit on time every night because she has streamlined her charting is far more motivated to try AI tools than a nurse who reads a policy about AI adoption. Be the demonstration before you worry about the mandate.

Common Roadblocks and Solutions

If the output is not good enough, the prompt is almost always too vague. Go back to Chapter 4 and rebuild the prompt with more specificity.

If your facility has not approved anything, focus on non-PHI tasks with general AI tools while you advocate for institutional adoption. Document the time you spend on documentation tasks and share that data with your manager.

If reviewing AI output feels like it takes as long as writing the note, the prompt is not producing output close enough to what you need. Invest time in improving the prompt during a less busy shift.

If AI made an error and now you do not trust it, that is actually the review process working. AI will make errors. The system you are building is designed to catch those errors before they enter the record. One error is a reason to pay attention to where that type of error occurs, not a reason to abandon the tool.

KEY TAKEAWAYS

- Start by finding out what your facility has approved before investing time in any AI tool.
- Phase 1 is practice on low-stakes tasks only. Phase 2 introduces real clinical tasks with a safety structure. Phase 3 builds consistent habits. Phase 4 is sustainable integration.
- Building a personal prompt library is the single most important long-term investment in AI integration.
- Common roadblocks all have specific solutions. None of them are reasons to abandon the practice.

Chapter 13
Case Studies

Case Study 1: The Med-Surg Nurse Who Got Her Evenings Back

Priya is a registered nurse with six years of experience on a busy medical-surgical unit. Her typical assignment is five patients per shift. Before AI, her end-of-shift charting averaged two hours after the shift officially ended.

She started with the handoff SBAR prompt from Appendix A during a relatively quiet stretch of shifts. Her first few attempts produced output that was structurally correct but missing qualitative information she had to add. Within two weeks she had modified the prompt to explicitly ask for the sections she always had to add, which reduced her post-output editing time significantly.

Three months in, her end-of-shift charting takes about thirty minutes for five patients. Her documentation quality also improved because the structured format consistently prompted her to include information she sometimes rushed through at the end of a long shift. The AI did not make her a better clinical nurse. But it made her documentation more consistently thorough.

Case Study 2: The ICU Team That Standardized Handoffs

Marcus is a charge nurse in a twelve-bed medical ICU. His unit had a longstanding problem with variable handoff quality. Some nurses gave exceptionally thorough handoffs. Others were more rushed and inconsistent. Information gaps between shifts were contributing to near-miss events.

He worked with his unit's clinical educator to develop a standardized SBAR handoff prompt specifically designed for the ICU context, with sections for hemodynamic status, ventilator parameters, drip management, and outstanding issues. Within two months the unit's handoff quality scores on their internal safety audit improved noticeably. The lesson: AI prompts used as organizational tools can improve consistency across a team, not just efficiency for individuals.

Case Study 3: The Pitfall of Trusting Output Without Review

Danielle is an experienced home health nurse with fifteen years in the field. After several weeks of good results, she began approving AI output with less thorough review on busy days. On one occasion, she submitted notes from two different patient visits in quick succession. A detail from the first patient's visit appeared in the second patient's note because her prompt input had inadvertently included information from both patients.

She caught it during her end-of-day review before submitting to the EHR, but only because she happened to notice something that did not fit. The lesson: AI documentation requires the same level of review on busy days as on slow days. The risk is not that AI makes more errors when you are busy. The risk is that you review less carefully when you are busy, which is exactly when errors are most likely to enter the record.

Case Study 4: The Nurse Practitioner Using a Hybrid Approach

Renata is a family nurse practitioner in an independent primary care practice. Her documentation burden includes full SOAP notes for patient encounters, referral letters, patient education materials, and prior authorization requests. Before AI integration, she regularly spent three to four hours after clinic hours on documentation.

She uses a HIPAA-compliant enterprise AI tool for her clinical documentation, a general AI tool for prior authorization letters and administrative correspondence that does not contain PHI, and her standard EHR templates for routine note elements that the AI tools did not improve. Her post-clinic documentation time has decreased to about ninety minutes. The lesson: for nurses in settings without institutional AI adoption, the individual compliance research is worth doing. The hybrid approach is a practical and compliant path forward.

KEY TAKEAWAYS

- AI documentation assistance can improve both efficiency and quality when implemented with attention to prompt design and consistent review habits.
- AI used as a standardization tool across a nursing team can reduce variation in documentation quality and decrease information gaps between shifts.
- The review step cannot be relaxed during busy periods. That is precisely when errors are most likely to enter the record if review is rushed.
- For nurses in settings without institutional AI adoption, a thoughtful hybrid approach using different tools for PHI and non-PHI tasks is a practical and compliant path forward.

Chapter 14

Burnout, Self-Care, and Long-Term Sustainability

What AI Can Actually Do for Nurse Burnout

Nurse burnout is not primarily a documentation problem. It is a systemic problem rooted in staffing ratios, organizational culture, healthcare system pressures, and working conditions. No AI tool can fix any of that.

What AI can do is return a portion of the hours that get consumed by administrative work, the hours that should be yours. If documentation is currently taking ninety minutes of your post-shift time and AI reduces that to thirty minutes, you have reclaimed an hour. Every shift. That is an hour of sleep, an hour with your family, an hour of decompression. Multiplied across a career, that is significant.

The research on burnout consistently identifies time pressure, cognitive load, and the sense of being unable to complete work within reasonable boundaries as the most significant contributors to emotional exhaustion. Reducing documentation time addresses all three.

Using AI for Nurse Self-Care and Reflection

Category 6 of the prompt library is the most personally oriented category in the book. Post-shift debrief prompts help you process the emotional weight of difficult shifts in a structured way. The framework they use is simple: what happened, what you felt, what you would do differently, and what you are taking away.

This kind of structured reflection is known to reduce the rumination that keeps nurses awake after difficult shifts and to support the emotional processing that prevents moral distress from accumulating over time. These prompts work best when you use them on difficult days. The instinct after a hard shift is often to avoid thinking about it. The reflection process is the opposite of that instinct, and it tends to produce better outcomes for emotional recovery.

Stress processing prompts help you articulate what is most weighing on you when everything feels heavy. Boundary-setting prompts help you draft professional communications for situations where you need to decline, push back, or raise a concern. Nurses are consistently socialized away from self-advocacy, and having language to work with can make a real difference.

The Cognitive Load Connection

One dimension of the burnout discussion that often gets overlooked is cognitive load. Burnout research consistently identifies cognitive overload as a separate and significant contributor to emotional exhaustion, distinct from time pressure alone. A nurse who is mentally exhausted from holding twelve hours of clinical details in her head while simultaneously trying to translate them into documentation language is experiencing a specific kind of depletion that time off does not fully address.

AI-assisted documentation reduces cognitive load in a specific way. When you know that your micro-notes will be organized and structured by a tool, you do not have to hold the entire shift in working memory. You can process each patient interaction and let it go, rather than mentally accumulating everything you will need to reconstruct later. Over a twelve-hour shift, that difference in working memory load is meaningful.

Nurses who have been using AI documentation tools for six months or more consistently report not just having more time, but feeling less mentally depleted at the end of shifts. The time savings are easier to measure. The cognitive load reduction is harder to quantify but may be equally significant for long-term sustainability in the profession.

Protecting the Time You Reclaim

The trap that some nurses fall into after AI integration is filling the reclaimed time with more work. Finishing charting in thirty minutes and then doing an extra hour of administrative tasks because they are now available is not the outcome this book is aiming for.

Before you integrate AI into your documentation workflow, decide what you are going to do with the time you reclaim. Sleep. Exercise. Be present with the people you care about. Pursue something that has nothing to do with nursing. Having a specific, valued use for reclaimed time is what makes the reduction in documentation time feel like a real benefit rather than an opportunity to do more work.

Nurse burnout will not be solved by AI. It will be solved by adequate staffing, fair compensation, functional organizational cultures, and systemic healthcare reform. What is in this book is a set of tools for the working nurse who needs to practice well and sustain herself today, while that larger work continues. You can use AI to reclaim your time and also advocate for the systemic changes that would prevent the documentation burden from existing in the first place. Both things are true. Both things are worth doing.

KEY TAKEAWAYS

- Documentation burden is one measurable, addressable contributor to nurse burnout. AI documentation assistance can return meaningful amounts of time per shift.
- Category 6 of the prompt library includes prompts for post-shift debrief, stress processing, and professional boundary-setting. These prompts are for the nurse, not for the chart.
- Protecting the time you reclaim is as important as reclaiming it. Having a specific, valued use for that time from the beginning of AI integration prevents it from being absorbed into more work.
- AI does not solve the systemic drivers of nurse burnout. Reducing documentation time is one tool among many, and it coexists with advocacy for systemic change.

Chapter 15
The Future of AI in Nursing

Five Trends Worth Watching

Ambient AI documentation will become the standard in well-resourced settings. The technology that listens to clinical encounters and produces structured documentation in real time is being adapted for nursing. When a nurse can walk out of a patient room with a documentation draft already generated from the conversation and assessment that just happened, the documentation burden shifts fundamentally.

EHR integration will deepen. The current generation of AI documentation assistance requires nurses to work in a separate tool and then transfer content to the EHR. The next generation will be integrated directly into the EHR workflow, making AI assistance invisible as a separate step.

AI-assisted clinical decision support will expand into nursing specifically. Nursing-specific tools that support triage assessment, early deterioration recognition, care planning, and risk stratification are in development and early deployment.

Regulatory clarity will develop. The regulatory environment around AI in healthcare is actively evolving. HIPAA guidance, state nursing practice acts, and accreditation standards are all developing more specific positions on AI use. Staying current with these developments is part of practicing with professional competence in the AI era.

The nursing profession will play a larger role in AI governance. The ANA's 2025 positioning on AI reflects a profession that is actively staking a claim in how AI is developed and deployed in healthcare. Nurses who understand AI and can speak credibly about its implications for clinical practice are increasingly valuable on technology governance committees and health system leadership bodies.

What Will Not Change

The ethical core of nursing will not change. Caring, compassion, advocacy, and the primacy of the patient relationship are the foundations of the profession regardless of what technology surrounds them. Technology must serve these values, not the other way around.

The need for clinical judgment will not change. AI will continue to get better at pattern recognition, at producing clinical language, and at structuring complex information. It will not get better at the kind of embodied, relational, intuitive knowing that comes from years at the bedside. That knowing is irreplaceable and it is what nursing actually is.

The accountability of the nurse will not change. The nurse who signs the documentation is responsible for it. This accountability is not a burden imposed on nurses by regulation. It is the expression of professional authority that makes nursing meaningful.

A Closing Vision

Maria Santos drove home before midnight.

Maria Santos whom we read about in Chapter 1 sat in her car in the driveway at nearly midnight, too tired to be hungry, running back through a twelve-hour shift to make sure she had documented everything. Six months later, the same nurse is charting in real time and finishing before she leaves the unit, getting home with enough energy left to be a person instead of just an exhausted professional.

That is not a small thing. Nursing is one of the most important professions in the world. The people who do it well are carrying a weight that most people who have never done it cannot fully understand. This book does not fix the larger problems. What it does is offer a set of tools for doing the work more sustainably. Tools that return hours. Tools that reduce the cognitive load of documentation so that more of your mental energy stays where it belongs: with your patients and with yourself.

You became a nurse because nursing matters. AI does not change what matters. It just gives you a little more of yourself to bring to it.

KEY TAKEAWAYS

- Ambient AI documentation, deeper EHR integration, nursing-specific clinical decision support, evolving regulatory clarity, and nursing's growing role in AI governance are the five most significant trends to watch.
- The ethical core of nursing, the requirement for clinical judgment, and the accountability of the nurse are constants that no amount of technological change will alter.
- Staying current without burnout requires following a small number of reliable nursing-specific sources and engaging with facility staff about AI adoption when opportunities arise.

Chapter 16

Appendix A: Complete Nursing Prompt Library - 60 Ready-to-Use Prompts

Each prompt is built on the master template from Chapter 5. Replace the bracketed sections with your anonymized clinical content. Always review output before use.

CATEGORY 1: Shift Preparation and Handoff Documentation (Prompts 1-14)

Prompt 1: Incoming Shift Patient Priority Assessment

You are a registered nurse beginning a new shift. Using the following anonymized patient summaries, create a prioritized patient list organized from highest to lowest clinical concern. For each patient, include a one-sentence status summary and one key action item for the start of the shift. Do not include patient names or identifiers. [Paste anonymous patient summaries here.] End with: [REQUIRES NURSE REVIEW AND CLINICAL VERIFICATION BEFORE USE]

Prompt 2: End-of-Shift SBAR Handoff - Single Patient

You are a registered nurse preparing an end-of-shift handoff. Using the following anonymized shift summary, write a complete SBAR handoff note. Include all four sections: Situation, Background, Assessment, and Recommendation. Use concise clinical language. Do not add information not present in the input. [Paste an anonymous shift summary here.] End with: [REQUIRES NURSE REVIEW AND CLINICAL VERIFICATION BEFORE USE]

Prompt 3: End-of-Shift SBAR Handoff - Full Patient Panel

You are a registered nurse preparing end-of-shift handoffs for multiple patients. For each anonymized patient summary provided, write a brief SBAR handoff. Keep each SBAR under 150 words. Organize output clearly by patient identifier. [Paste anonymized summaries for each patient, labeled Patient A, Patient B, etc.] End with: [REQUIRES NURSE REVIEW AND CLINICAL VERIFICATION BEFORE USE]

Prompt 4: Admission Handoff Receiving Summary

You are a registered nurse receiving a new admission. Using the following anonymized admission information, create an organized admission receiving summary that includes: chief complaint, relevant history, current vital signs, active orders and scheduled medications, immediate priorities, and outstanding tasks. [Paste anonymous admission data.] End with: [REQUIRES NURSE REVIEW AND CLINICAL VERIFICATION BEFORE USE]

Prompt 5: Transfer Handoff - Unit to Unit

You are a registered nurse preparing a transfer handoff summary for a patient moving to another unit. Write a complete transfer summary including: reason for transfer, current clinical status, active medications, recent procedures or interventions, outstanding orders, and priority information for the receiving unit. [Paste an anonymous clinical summary.] End with: [REQUIRES NURSE REVIEW AND CLINICAL VERIFICATION BEFORE USE]

Prompt 6: Pre-Procedure Preparation Checklist

You are a registered nurse preparing a patient for a procedure. Based on the following anonymized patient information and procedure type, create a pre-procedure nursing checklist covering: patient verification requirements, consent status, NPO status, IV access, lab values to verify, allergies confirmation, vital sign baseline, and patient education points. [Paste anonymized patient and procedure information.] End with: [REQUIRES NURSE REVIEW AND CLINICAL VERIFICATION BEFORE USE]

Prompt 7: Discharge Planning Summary

You are a registered nurse preparing a patient for discharge. Using the following anonymized clinical information, write a discharge planning summary that includes: discharge status, medications to go home, follow-up appointments needed, patient education completed, patient's demonstrated understanding, support system, and any outstanding items before discharge can be completed. [Paste anonymized information.] End with: [REQUIRES NURSE REVIEW AND CLINICAL VERIFICATION BEFORE USE]

Prompt 8: Shift Report for Night to Day Transition

You are a night shift nurse preparing a morning handoff to the day team. Write a structured overnight summary that covers: patient status at start of night, significant overnight events or changes, vital sign trends, medication administration, any calls made to providers and orders received, sleep and comfort status, and morning priorities. [Paste anonymous overnight summary.] End with: [REQUIRES NURSE REVIEW AND CLINICAL VERIFICATION BEFORE USE]

Prompt 9: Rapid Response or Emergency Handoff

You are a registered nurse preparing an urgent handoff after a rapid response or emergency situation. Write a concise SBAR summary focused on: what happened, the patient's current status, interventions performed and patient response, current orders and monitoring in place, and what needs to happen in the next hour. Keep the summary under 100 words. [Paste anonymous event summary.] End with: [REQUIRES NURSE REVIEW AND CLINICAL VERIFICATION BEFORE USE]

Prompt 10: End-of-Shift Summary for Charge Nurse

You are a registered nurse preparing an end-of-shift summary for your charge nurse. Summarize the shift status of your patient panel, noting any significant events, current patient acuity concerns, outstanding orders or tasks, family communication needs, and anything the charge nurse needs to know for staffing or resource purposes. [Paste an anonymous patient panel summary.] End with: [REQUIRES NURSE REVIEW AND CLINICAL VERIFICATION BEFORE USE]

Prompt 11: Care Conference Preparation Summary

You are a registered nurse preparing for an interdisciplinary care conference. Write a nursing summary for each patient on the conference agenda, covering: current status, nursing priorities, patient and family concerns, progress toward care goals, discharge barriers, and nursing recommendations for the conference. [Paste anonymized patient information.] End with: [REQUIRES NURSE REVIEW AND CLINICAL VERIFICATION BEFORE USE]

Prompt 12: Float Nurse Orientation Summary

You are a charge nurse orienting a float or agency nurse to your unit's current patient panel. Write a brief, organized orientation summary for each patient that covers: diagnosis and reason for admission, current status and acuity level, key nursing care priorities, any alerts or safety concerns, and one specific instruction for each patient's care. [Paste anonymous patient panel information.] End with: [REQUIRES NURSE REVIEW AND CLINICAL VERIFICATION BEFORE USE]

Prompt 13: Weekend Handoff - Long-Gap Summary

You are a nurse preparing a handoff summary for a nurse who will be caring for your patients over a weekend or extended period. Write a comprehensive summary for each patient that provides enough context for a nurse who has not cared for them before, including relevant background, current status, plan of care, anticipated changes, and contact information for covering providers. [Paste anonymized patient information.] End with: [REQUIRES NURSE REVIEW AND CLINICAL VERIFICATION BEFORE USE]

Prompt 14: Patient Assignment Acceptance Documentation

You are a registered nurse documenting your acceptance of a patient assignment at the start of shift. Write a brief assignment acceptance note confirming the patients accepted, any concerns noted about the assignment, any equipment or safety issues identified, and any deferred tasks from the outgoing nurse. [Paste anonymous assignment information.] End with: [REQUIRES NURSE REVIEW AND CLINICAL VERIFICATION BEFORE USE]

CATEGORY 2: Clinical Notes and Charting (Prompts 15-27)

Prompt 15: SOAP Note - General Assessment

You are a registered nurse writing a SOAP assessment note. Using the following anonymized clinical data, write a complete SOAP note with clearly labeled sections for Subjective, Objective, Assessment, and Plan. Use past tense. Use objective clinical language. Do not add clinical information not present in the input. [Paste anonymized assessment data.] End with: [REQUIRES NURSE REVIEW AND CLINICAL VERIFICATION BEFORE USE]

Prompt 16: DAR Note - General

You are a registered nurse writing a DAR documentation note. Using the following anonymized clinical information, write a DAR note with clearly labeled Data, Action, and Response sections. Keep each section focused and clinically specific. [Paste anonymized clinical information.] End with: [REQUIRES NURSE REVIEW AND CLINICAL VERIFICATION BEFORE USE]

Prompt 17: PIE Note

You are a registered nurse writing a PIE nursing note. Using the following anonymized clinical information, write a PIE note with clearly labeled Problem, Intervention, and Evaluation sections. Identify the specific nursing problem being addressed in the Problem section. [Paste anonymized information.] End with: [REQUIRES NURSE REVIEW AND CLINICAL VERIFICATION BEFORE USE]

Prompt 18: Focus Charting Note

You are a registered nurse writing a Focus Charting note. The focus for this note is [state focus: e.g., pain management, respiratory status, mobility]. Write a DAR note centered on this focus, using only the following anonymized clinical data. [Paste anonymized data relevant to the focus.] End with: [REQUIRES NURSE REVIEW AND CLINICAL VERIFICATION BEFORE USE]

Prompt 19: Post-Procedure Assessment Note

You are a registered nurse documenting a post-procedure assessment. Write a structured post-procedure nursing note that covers: time of return from procedure, patient's level of consciousness and orientation, vital signs, pain assessment, site assessment, IV access status, any immediate post-procedure concerns, and nursing plan. [Paste anonymized post-procedure assessment data.] End with: [REQUIRES NURSE REVIEW AND CLINICAL VERIFICATION BEFORE USE]

Prompt 20: Fall Risk and Safety Assessment

You are a registered nurse documenting a fall risk and safety assessment. Write a structured safety note that covers: fall risk score and contributing factors, current fall prevention measures in place, patient and family education provided, environmental safety measures, and nursing plan for fall prevention. [Paste anonymized safety assessment data.] End with: [REQUIRES NURSE REVIEW AND CLINICAL VERIFICATION BEFORE USE]

Prompt 21: Pain Assessment and Management Note

You are a registered nurse documenting pain assessment and management. Write a clinical pain management note covering: pain location and character as reported by the patient, numeric pain rating, aggravating and relieving factors, medications administered and times, non-pharmacological interventions used, and patient's response to treatment. [Paste anonymized pain assessment data.] End with: [REQUIRES NURSE REVIEW AND CLINICAL VERIFICATION BEFORE USE]

Prompt 22: Skin Assessment and Wound Note

You are a registered nurse documenting a skin assessment and wound evaluation. Write a structured skin and wound note covering: overall skin integrity assessment, wound location and description including size, depth, tissue type, drainage, and edges, wound care performed, patient response, and nursing plan for wound management. [Paste anonymized assessment data.] End with: [REQUIRES NURSE REVIEW AND CLINICAL VERIFICATION BEFORE USE]

Prompt 23: Respiratory Assessment Note

You are a registered nurse documenting a respiratory assessment. Write a structured respiratory note covering: respiratory rate, depth, and effort, lung sounds on auscultation, oxygen saturation and supplemental oxygen if applicable, sputum characteristics if applicable, patient's subjective report, and respiratory interventions performed. [Paste anonymized assessment data.] End with: [REQUIRES NURSE REVIEW AND CLINICAL VERIFICATION BEFORE USE]

Prompt 24: Neurovascular Assessment Note

You are a registered nurse documenting a neurovascular assessment for an extremity. Write a structured neurovascular note covering: skin color and temperature, capillary refill time, sensation, movement, pulse quality, pain with passive stretch if applicable, and comparison to the unaffected extremity. [Paste anonymized assessment data.] End with: [REQUIRES NURSE REVIEW AND CLINICAL VERIFICATION BEFORE USE]

Prompt 25: Behavioral Health Assessment Note

You are a registered nurse documenting a behavioral health nursing assessment. Write a structured behavioral health note covering: appearance and behavior, affect and mood as observed and reported, thought process and content, orientation and cognition, safety assessment, current medications and compliance, and nursing plan. Do not include diagnostic conclusions. [Paste anonymized assessment data.] End with: [REQUIRES NURSE REVIEW AND CLINICAL VERIFICATION BEFORE USE]

Prompt 26: Discharge Note

You are a registered nurse writing a discharge documentation note. Write a structured discharge note covering: condition at time of discharge, discharge destination, mode of transport, medications dispensed or prescriptions given, education provided and patient's demonstrated understanding, follow-up appointments, and signature confirmation elements. [Paste anonymous discharge summary.] End with: [REQUIRES NURSE REVIEW AND CLINICAL VERIFICATION BEFORE USE]

Prompt 27: Incident or Event Note

You are a registered nurse documenting a clinical event or near-miss incident. Write a factual, chronological event note covering: time the event was discovered, description of what was found, immediate nursing response and actions taken, patient's condition and response, notifications made and to whom and when, and current patient status. Use objective, factual language only. [Paste anonymous event information.] End with: [REQUIRES NURSE REVIEW AND CLINICAL VERIFICATION BEFORE USE]

CATEGORY 3: Care Planning and Goal Setting (Prompts 28-34)

Prompt 28: Nursing Care Plan - Three Priority Diagnoses

You are a registered nurse developing a nursing care plan. Based on the following anonymized patient information, identify three priority nursing diagnoses. For each diagnosis, write one SMART goal measurable within 48 hours and three evidence-based nursing interventions. [Paste anonymized patient information.] End with: [REQUIRES NURSE REVIEW AND CLINICAL VERIFICATION BEFORE USE]

Prompt 29: SMART Goal Development

You are a registered nurse writing measurable patient care goals. Using the following anonymized clinical information, write three SMART goals that are specific, measurable, achievable, relevant, and time-bound. Each goal should address a different nursing priority area. Specify the measurement criteria and the timeframe for each goal. [Paste anonymized clinical information.] End with: [REQUIRES NURSE REVIEW AND CLINICAL VERIFICATION BEFORE USE]

Prompt 30: Care Plan Update

You are a registered nurse updating an existing nursing care plan. Based on the following anonymized information about the patient's current status and progress, revise the care plan goals and interventions to reflect current clinical priorities. Note which previous goals have been met, which require modification, and any new priorities. [Paste anonymized current status information.] End with: [REQUIRES NURSE REVIEW AND CLINICAL VERIFICATION BEFORE USE]

Prompt 31: Interdisciplinary Care Conference Goals

You are a registered nurse preparing nursing goals for an interdisciplinary care conference. Write three to five nursing-specific goals for the conference that address the patient's primary nursing priorities, are measurable, include a target timeline, and specify the nursing team's role in achieving them. [Paste anonymized patient information.] End with: [REQUIRES NURSE REVIEW AND CLINICAL VERIFICATION BEFORE USE]

Prompt 32: Mobility and Rehabilitation Care Plan

You are a registered nurse writing a mobility and rehabilitation care plan component. Based on the following anonymized information about the patient's current mobility status, write SMART mobility goals for 24 hours, 48 hours, and discharge. Include specific nursing interventions for each goal. [Paste anonymized mobility assessment information.] End with: [REQUIRES NURSE REVIEW AND CLINICAL VERIFICATION BEFORE USE]

Prompt 33: Pain Management Care Plan

You are a registered nurse writing a pain management component of the nursing care plan. Based on the following anonymized pain assessment information, write a comprehensive pain management plan including: assessment schedule, pharmacological interventions, non-pharmacological interventions, goal pain scores, and criteria for escalating pain management. [Paste anonymized pain information.] End with: [REQUIRES NURSE REVIEW AND CLINICAL VERIFICATION BEFORE USE]

Prompt 34: Fall Prevention Care Plan

You are a registered nurse writing a fall prevention care plan. Based on the following anonymized fall risk assessment, write a comprehensive fall prevention plan including: environmental modifications, equipment needs, staff interventions, patient and family education, and monitoring schedule. [Paste anonymized fall risk information.] End with: [REQUIRES NURSE REVIEW AND CLINICAL VERIFICATION BEFORE USE]

CATEGORY 4: Patient Education Materials (Prompts 35-44)

Prompt 35: Medication Teaching Handout

You are a registered nurse creating a patient medication education handout. Write a clear, plain-language guide for a patient starting a new medication. Use a 6th grade reading level. Include: what this medication is for in plain language, how to take it correctly, common side effects to expect, serious side effects requiring immediate medical attention, and foods or other medications to avoid. [Specify medication type and any relevant patient context.] End with a brief summary checklist.

Prompt 36: Discharge Instructions - General

You are a registered nurse writing discharge instructions for a patient going home. Write clear, patient-friendly discharge instructions that cover: activity restrictions, diet instructions, wound or procedure care if applicable, medications, warning signs requiring a call to the provider, warning signs requiring emergency care, and scheduled follow-up. Use a 6th grade reading level. [Specify condition and relevant patient discharge context.]

Prompt 37: Wound Care Home Instructions

You are a registered nurse creating home wound care instructions for a patient being discharged. Write step-by-step instructions for wound care at home, including: supplies needed, hand hygiene instructions, wound cleaning procedure, dressing change instructions, signs of infection to watch for, and when to call the provider. Use simple numbered steps and plain language. [Specify wound type if relevant.]

Prompt 38: Chronic Disease Self-Management Guide

You are a registered nurse creating a self-management education guide for a patient with a chronic condition. Write a clear, practical guide covering: understanding the condition in plain language, daily self-monitoring recommendations, lifestyle modifications, medication management, when to call the provider, and one simple daily habit that supports management. Use a 6th grade reading level. [Specify condition.]

Prompt 39: Pre-Procedure Patient Education

You are a registered nurse creating patient education for an upcoming procedure. Write a patient-friendly explanation covering: what the procedure is and why it is needed in plain language, how to prepare including diet, medication, and activity instructions, what to expect during the procedure, what recovery looks like, and questions the patient should ask their provider. [Specify procedure type.]

Prompt 40: Post-Operative Care Instructions

You are a registered nurse writing post-operative care instructions for a patient after a surgical procedure. Cover: activity restrictions, incision care, pain management instructions, diet progression, when to resume normal activities, signs of complications to watch for, and follow-up instructions. Use plain language and numbered steps where appropriate. [Specify surgery type and any relevant patient factors.]

Prompt 41: Pediatric Care Instructions for Parents

You are a registered nurse writing care instructions for the parents of a pediatric patient. Write clear, reassuring instructions for home care that cover: the child's condition in plain language appropriate for a parent, what normal recovery looks like, specific care tasks, warning signs requiring immediate attention, and when and how to contact the provider. Use warm, accessible language. [Specify the child's condition and age range.]

Prompt 42: Dietary Education Handout

You are a registered nurse creating a dietary education handout. Write a simple, practical guide covering: why dietary changes are important for this patient's condition, specific foods to include more of, specific foods to limit or avoid, practical meal planning tips, and a sample one-day meal plan. Use a 6th grade reading level. [Specify dietary restriction type.]

Prompt 43: Activity and Exercise Instructions

You are a registered nurse writing activity and exercise guidelines for a patient following discharge or diagnosis. Write clear instructions covering: current activity restrictions and why they exist, safe activities the patient can do, a gradual return-to-activity plan, warning signs to stop and rest, and when to follow up before increasing activity. [Specify condition and activity level context.]

Prompt 44: Mental Health Self-Care Guide for Patients

You are a registered nurse creating a patient mental health self-care guide. Write a supportive, plain-language guide covering: simple daily self-care practices, stress management techniques, sleep hygiene recommendations, when to reach out to a provider or support person, and crisis resources. Use warm, non-clinical language. Avoid diagnostic labels.

CATEGORY 5: Between-Shift and Administrative Support (Prompts 45-50)

Prompt 45: Professional Email to Provider

You are a registered nurse drafting a professional communication to a provider. Write a clear, direct email that follows SBAR structure. State the reason for the communication in the first sentence. Be specific about what information you need or what action you are requesting. Maintain a professional, collaborative tone. [Describe the situation and what you need from the provider.]

Prompt 46: Patient Safety Concern Communication

You are a registered nurse drafting a professional communication about a patient safety concern. Write a clear, factual communication that describes the safety concern specifically, explains the potential impact on patient care, states what you have already done, and requests a specific response or action. Use objective, professional language. [Describe the safety concern and context.]

Prompt 47: Shift Incident Report Preparation

You are a registered nurse preparing documentation for an incident report. Write a chronological factual summary of the following event that includes: date and time, description of what occurred, persons involved by role only, immediate actions taken, current status, and follow-up actions needed. Use objective language only. [Describe the incident using anonymized information.]

Prompt 48: Competency and Professional Development Documentation

You are a registered nurse documenting a professional development activity or competency demonstration. Write a structured reflection that covers: what the activity or competency was, what you learned or demonstrated, how you will apply it in practice, and the date and context of completion. [Describe the development activity or competency.]

Prompt 49: Policy or Protocol Clarification Request

You are a registered nurse drafting a request for policy clarification. Write a professional email requesting specific clarification on a nursing policy or protocol. State the specific policy or situation in question, explain why clarity is needed, and request a specific response. Keep it brief and focused. [Describe the policy question and context.]

Prompt 50: Committee or Meeting Preparation Summary

You are a registered nurse preparing for a committee meeting or professional meeting. Write a brief preparation summary covering: the purpose of the meeting, key agenda items relevant to nursing, information or data you should bring, questions or concerns you want to raise, and your desired outcome from the meeting. [Describe the meeting and relevant context.]

CATEGORY 6: Nurse Self-Care and Reflection (Prompts 51-60)

Prompt 51: Post-Shift Debrief

You are a supportive clinical reflection facilitator. Ask me five structured questions to help me process today's nursing shift. After I answer, provide a brief organized reflection summary. Focus on: what went well, what was challenging, what I would do differently, what I learned, and one thing I am doing to take care of myself tonight. Begin with the first question now.

Prompt 52: Critical Incident Processing

You are a supportive clinical reflection guide. Help me process a difficult or emotionally significant clinical situation using a structured reflection framework. Ask me about what happened, my clinical response, my emotional response, whether I would change anything, and what support I need. Ask one question at a time. Begin now.

Prompt 53: Moral Distress Reflection

You are a supportive professional reflection guide. I experienced a situation today that created moral distress, it was a conflict between what I believed was right and what I was able to do. Help me articulate the conflict, identify what I could and could not control, and think about healthy ways to process this experience. Ask me guiding questions one at a time.

Prompt 54: End-of-Week Professional Reflection

You are a supportive professional development guide. Ask me five questions to help me reflect on my nursing practice this week. Cover: a moment I am proud of, a challenge I faced and how I handled it, something I learned, a way I supported a colleague, and one professional goal for next week. Ask one question at a time.

Prompt 55: Compassion Fatigue Self-Assessment

You are a supportive wellness guide. Ask me a series of reflective questions to help me assess my current level of compassion fatigue and identify specific areas where I need support or self-care. Be compassionate and non-judgmental in your approach. Ask one question at a time and respond to each answer before asking the next.

Prompt 56: Setting Professional Boundaries

You are a professional communication coach. Help me draft a clear, professional response to the following workplace situation where I need to set a limit or decline a request. The response should be direct, respectful, and specific about what I can and cannot do. [Describe the situation.]

Prompt 57: Difficult Conversation Preparation

You are a communication coach for healthcare professionals. Help me prepare for a difficult conversation I need to have at work. Ask me about the situation, what I hope to achieve, my concerns about the conversation, and what I need from the other person. Then help me draft an opening statement that is direct, professional, and non-confrontational.

Prompt 58: Career Development Reflection

You are a nursing career development guide. Ask me a series of questions to help me reflect on where I am in my nursing career, what I value most in my work, what I want to develop, and what my next professional steps might be. Ask one question at a time.

Prompt 59: Gratitude and Meaning Practice

You are a reflective practice guide. Ask me three to five questions designed to help me identify moments of meaning, connection, and accomplishment from my recent nursing work. Help me articulate what made those moments significant. This practice is about reconnecting with why nursing matters to me.

Prompt 60: Return-to-Work Preparation After Time Off

You are a supportive transition guide. I am returning to clinical nursing after a period away. Ask me questions to help me identify any anxiety or concerns about returning, any knowledge or skill areas I want to review before my first shift, and practical steps I can take to feel prepared and confident. Ask one question at a time.

Chapter 17

Appendix B: Ethical Checklist and Compliance Templates

B.1: Pre-Use AI Checklist for Nursing Documentation

Use this checklist before submitting any clinical prompt or using any AI output in patient care.

Before Submitting the Prompt

- I have removed all patient names, dates of birth, room numbers, and medical record numbers from my input
- The AI tool I am using has been approved by my facility, or I am using a compliant tool for non-facility use
- My prompt specifies the role, task, format, and relevant constraints
- My prompt includes an instruction to end with the human review reminder
- The task I am asking AI to perform is within appropriate use boundaries

Before Using the AI Output

- I have read the entire output from beginning to end
- Every clinical statement in the output is accurate and reflects my clinical assessment
- I have added any qualitative observations or clinical detail that is missing from the output
- I have removed any content that does not apply to this patient
- The output does not contain any PHI that should not be in the documentation
- I am prepared to sign my name to this documentation and take full professional responsibility for its accuracy

B.2: Facility AI Use Disclosure Template

Use this template when discussing AI use with patients who ask, or when your facility requires documentation of AI-assisted care elements.

TEMPLATE: This facility uses AI-assisted tools to support nursing documentation and patient education materials. All documentation and materials produced with AI assistance are reviewed, verified, and approved by your nursing care team before being used in your care or placed in your medical record. Your nurse remains fully responsible for all aspects of your care and documentation.

B.3: Personal Practice AI Policy Template

Adapt this template as your personal practice policy for AI use in your nursing work.

- I will use AI documentation assistance only with HIPAA-compliant tools approved for clinical use, or with complete anonymization of all patient information when using general tools for non-PHI tasks.

- I will review every AI output completely before using it in patient care, entering it into any clinical record, or sharing it with any other member of the care team.

- I will correct all errors, add all missing clinical information, and remove all inapplicable content from every AI output before signing my name to it.

- I will not use AI to perform clinical assessment, make clinical decisions, or substitute for my professional judgment in any area of nursing practice.

- I will stay informed about my facility's policies on AI use and will update my practice as those policies evolve.

Chapter 18

Appendix C: Glossary of AI and Nursing Terms

Ambient documentation: AI technology that listens to clinical conversations or encounters and automatically generates structured documentation without requiring manual input by the nurse.

Artificial intelligence (AI): A category of computer technology that uses algorithms to perform tasks that typically require human intelligence, including language understanding, pattern recognition, and content generation.

Business Associate Agreement (BAA): A legal contract between a healthcare organization and a vendor or service provider who handles Protected Health Information, establishing the vendor's responsibility for protecting that information under HIPAA.

EHR (Electronic Health Record): A digital version of a patient's medical chart, used for documentation, order management, and care coordination across a healthcare organization.

Hallucination: A term used in AI to describe the phenomenon of an AI language model generating confident, fluent, plausible-sounding content that is factually incorrect or not present in the input provided.

HIPAA: The Health Insurance Portability and Accountability Act. Federal legislation governing the use, storage, and transmission of Protected Health Information. All clinical AI use must comply with HIPAA requirements.

Large language model (LLM): The type of AI technology underlying tools like ChatGPT, Claude, and Gemini. LLMs are trained on large amounts of text data and are capable of generating human-like language, answering questions, and producing structured written content.

PHI (Protected Health Information): Any individually identifiable health information held or transmitted by a covered entity. Includes names, dates, geographic identifiers, phone numbers, and any other information that could be used to identify a specific patient in connection with their health status or care.

Prompt: The instruction given to an AI tool that describes what the user wants the tool to produce. The quality of the prompt is the primary determinant of the quality of the AI output.

Prompt engineering: The practice of constructing prompts in ways that consistently produce accurate, useful, and appropriately formatted AI output. A learnable skill that improves with practice.

SBAR: Situation, Background, Assessment, Recommendation. A structured communication framework widely used in healthcare for patient handoffs, provider communication, and clinical summaries.

Chapter 19

Appendix D: Resources and Further Reading

Professional Guidelines

- ANA Code of Ethics for Nurses (2025): codeofethics.ana.org
- ANA Position Statement: The Ethical Use of Artificial Intelligence in Nursing Practice (2022, revised 2025): Published in OJIN: The Online Journal of Issues in Nursing, Volume 30, Number 2, May 2025
- American Academy of Nursing AI Policy Priorities 2025-2026: aannet.org

HIPAA and Compliance

- HHS Office for Civil Rights HIPAA guidance: hhs.gov/hipaa
- HHS guidance on AI and HIPAA: hhs.gov/hipaa - search for AI guidance updates

Nursing Organizations

- American Nurses Association: nursingworld.org
- National Council of State Boards of Nursing: ncsbn.org
- Specialty nursing organization websites for discipline-specific AI guidance

Stay Current

The best source for tools and policies specific to your practice environment are your facility's nursing informatics team. Ask to be included in communications about AI adoption and updates. For ongoing learning about AI in healthcare and nursing, monitor publications from your specialty nursing organization, the ANA's continuing education offerings, and peer-reviewed journals in your clinical area.

★ ★ ★ ★ ★

Thank You for Reading!

We hope you enjoyed this book and found value in its content. Please consider leaving an honest review. It takes just a minute. Reviews are so important to independent publishers.

LEAVE A REVIEW

Made in the USA
Monee, IL
04 May 2026

49473130R00070